Finding Your Smile Again

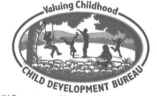

Valuing Childhood

CHILD DEVELOPMENT BUREAU

NH Department of Health and Human Services
Division for Children, Youth and Families
1-800-852-3345 x 4451

Other Books by Jeff A. Johnson

Do-It-Yourself Early Learning:
Easy and Fun Activities and Toys from
Everyday Home Center Materials

Finding Your Smile Again

A Child Care Professional's Guide to Reducing Stress and Avoiding Burnout

Jeff A. Johnson

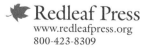
Redleaf Press
www.redleafpress.org
800-423-8309

Published by Redleaf Press
a division of Resources for Child Caring
10 Yorkton Court
St. Paul, MN 55117
Visit us online at www.redleafpress.org.

First edition 2007
Cover design by Amy Kirkpatrick
Cover photograph by Steve Wewerka
Interior typeset in 11/15 Goudy Old Style and designed by Prism Publishing Center
Interior illustrations by Kara Fellows
Printed in the United States of America
14 13 12 11 10 09 08 07   1 2 3 4 5 6 7 8

Redleaf Press books are available at a special discount when purchased in bulk
for special premiums and sales promotions. For details, contact the sales manager
at 800-423-8309.

Library of Congress Cataloging-in-Publication Data
Johnson, Jeff A., 1969–
    Finding your smile again : a child care professional's guide to reducing stress and
    avoiding burnout / Jeff A. Johnson.—1st ed.
        p. cm.
    Includes bibliographical references.
    ISBN 978-1-929610-93-8
    1. Child care workers—Job stress—United States. 2. Burn out (Psychology)—
Prevention. 3. Stress management. I. Title.
    HQ778.63.J64 2006
    362.701'9—dc22
                                                    2006038896

Printed on 30 percent postconsumer-waste recycled paper.

to Tasha,

my One True Love

Finding Your Smile Again

Foreword

THIS BOOK IS DESIGNED for people who have dedicated themselves to making the world of children and their families a better place. People work in the field of early care and education because they see that their caregiving and commitment just might make a difference in a crazy world.

The topic of burnout is one of great importance because many of us in this field give so much of ourselves to others that we have nothing left, either for ourselves or for those who are closest to us. Jeff invites readers into his life as he explains firsthand what he and his wife went through while they were burning out and then rebuilding their relationship. More important, Jeff shares how he and his wife, Tasha, decided to make changes so that they could continue to do the work both of them loved—working with children and their families.

Throughout the book, Jeff emphasizes that burnout can affect anyone who works in the field of early care and education: the family child care provider who works alone in her business; the center director who feels overwhelmed by staff, parents, children, and regulators coming at her on a daily basis; the teacher who feels unappreciated and underpaid; the Head Start educator who is overwhelmed by paperwork and governmental regulations. *Finding Your Smile Again* is written in an easy-to-read style that speaks directly to the daily experiences of this wide range of child care professionals and offers supportive suggestions that can be applied today. Most people who are dealing with burnout do not have time to sit down and read a book cover-to-cover before it can offer them any benefits. This book is different. You can pick it up, read a few pages or a chapter, and decide as you go what changes you need to make to feel better about your personal and professional life.

Jeff's sense of humor resonates throughout the book, and since humor is a coping mechanism that helps all of us immensely during stress and burnout, *Finding Your Smile Again* will lift your spirits and give you hope that there is a way out of feeling overwhelmed. (If you ever get the chance to hear Jeff's workshop on burnout at a conference, please go. You will not only leave feeling motivated and regenerated, but you will also find reinforcement for what you have learned in this book. This is how I felt after hearing Jeff's presentation and then reading *Finding Your Smile Again*.)

When you take care of yourself, you will be better able to take care of others. Everyone benefits! So sit back, relax, and take care of yourself by reading and enjoying *Finding Your Smile Again*. Go ahead. You deserve it!

—**Sue Baldwin**
INSIGHTS Training & Consulting

Go to www.suebaldwin.com to read about the books Sue has written for child care professionals and to learn about the trainings she offers.

Acknowledgments

THANKS TO Sonny Kellen for giving me the best job anyone could ever burn out at. You provided me with opportunities to succeed and screw up. You taught me how to do both with grace—and I learned oodles along the way. We both burned out, but we had a lot of fun and did heaps of good before it happened.

Thanks to Chris Blades for introducing me to yoga and meditation. Surviving burnout and writing this book were a great deal easier because you helped me learn to focus intently and let go completely at the same time.

Thanks to Goodwill Industries in Sioux City, Iowa, for providing a hideaway where I could write and not feel guilty. Your camp was a perfect place to get away from my to-do list and other distractions so I could write.

Thanks to the hundreds of early childhood professionals I've talked to about stress and burnout over the last few years. Many of the stories, ideas, and insights you've shared worked their way into this book. Michelle Gordon, Shanna Barton, Nikki Darling-Kuria, members of the Family Child Care Professionals of South Dakota, Angie Sewalson, Pam Stefanich, and Jim Davis: your help was invaluable.

Special thanks to Vicki Harris and Daphne Cole for helping Tasha and me transition from a state of burnout into family child care professionals.

Special thanks also to everyone at Redleaf Press who sculpted and refined my ideas and words into a real book.

Introduction

BACK WHEN THIS BOOK was just a hazy blur of ideas, I talked with Redleaf Press's editor-in-chief, Sid Farrar, about whether the book should focus solely on burnout among family-based providers or address the concerns of all early childhood professionals. We wondered if there were too many differences among early care and education programs and professionals for one book to deal with them all effectively. After some discussion, we finally agreed that when it comes to burnout, there are more similarities than differences. It doesn't matter if you work as a center director, lead teacher, classroom assistant, or cook. It doesn't matter if you own or work in a family child care program. It doesn't matter if you work in a preschool, Head Start program, or elementary school. Nor does it matter if your facility is brand spanking new or one hundred years old, or if this is your first week as a provider or you've been on the job for more than thirty years. If you are feeling stressed out, run-down, anxious, out of gas, over the edge, befuddled, broken, lost, astray, overwrought, uptight, drained, in a rut, in a rush, in a funk, or insignificant, this book can help.

We all have at least one thing in common: we are caregivers. And not just at work, either. Most of us habitually take care of other people. We are empathetic, giving, warm, and nurturing—and we have a hard time saying no to anyone who needs taking care of. We take care of not only children but also their families, our own families, our neighbors, our religious and civic groups, total strangers, stray dogs, and baby birds who have fallen from their nests. It's what we do.

◄ 1

The problem is the part about not being able to say *no*. When I train caregivers on the topic of burnout, I urge them to say *no* at least occasionally. In every session, a provider says, "I can't say *no*." We want to, we know it will unburden us, but we can't make the tiny and powerful word come out of our mouths. We feel guilty. It's as if we are letting someone down. Too often, we equate saying *no* with being weak or failing. So every request we hear gets a resounding *yes*.

"Can my kids stay an extra hour?" *Yes*.

"I can't pay you until next Wednesday, is that okay?" *Yes*.

"The baby has a fever—can you still watch her?" *Yes*.

"Mom, can I have $20?" *Yes*.

"It's Monday, and Maggie didn't show up again. Can you cover her hours?" *Yes*.

"Our licensing visit is next week; can you come in this weekend and do some cleaning so the place will be ready?" *Yes*.

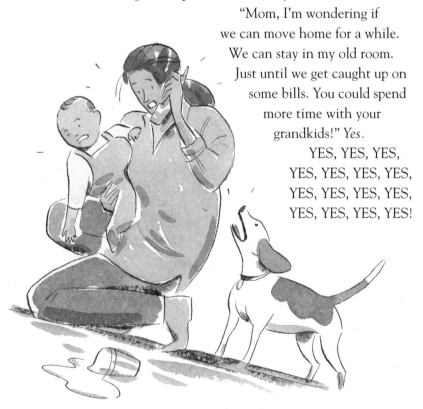

"Mom, I'm wondering if we can move home for a while. We can stay in my old room. Just until we get caught up on some bills. You could spend more time with your grandkids!" *Yes*.

YES, YES, YES, YES, YES, YES, YES, YES, YES, YES, YES, YES, YES, YES, YES!

We take care of everyone but ourselves. We give so much of our time and energy and so much of ourselves to others that we tend to neglect our own needs. We vainly try to hold things together, turning a strong face toward the world while falling apart inside. We need to ask ourselves: What is really happening here? Why are we sacrificing our physical and emotional health to the demands of a job?

If we choose to ignore our needs, no matter what our profession, we become physically and emotionally exhausted; we become burned out. This is what burnout looks like: We become detached from ourselves and from others; we become zombies who go through the motions of caregiving. Our hearts and minds are no longer in the work; we are out of tune. Burnout affects us physically as well: insomnia, sore backs and necks and knees, headaches, tight chests, queasy stomachs, and lack of energy. Burnout also affects us emotionally: we drift without focus or direction, filled with an all-consuming emptiness or anxiety and a variety of uneasy feelings. We neglect our families and friends, our coworkers and peers, and the children in our care because we lack the energy to deal with the myriad things we have said *yes* to. And here lies the irony of our situation: *the more we neglect our own needs to give to others, the more we shortchange them and ourselves.*

We need to care for ourselves first before we can care for others. This bears repeating. We need to care for ourselves first in order to have *the internal resources* to care for others. When we don't care for ourselves, personal dreams drift away into the dark corners of our minds. Goals go unrealized. Life becomes an unending slog through waist-deep mud.

When burnout reaches this point, we find ourselves at an important crossroads where we can choose to leave the profession entirely; make superficial changes (like a lateral job change) and continue as a burned-out zombie; or make subtle and mindful changes that lead in a fresh, energized, and positive direction. We have to choose our course and find our answers; no one can do it for us.

If you are still reading, you probably work as an early care and education professional. It doesn't matter where you work: child care center; preschool; Head Start or family child care program; elementary school; agency providing support for direct-care providers; or in someone else's home as a nanny, au pair, or caregiver to a relative. Wherever you fit into the early care and education field, you have at least some experience with burnout—if not your own, then that of a colleague. It's no wonder: We child care professionals have a lot on our shoulders. We have a huge social and economic impact on our community, our state, and our nation.

Imagine the havoc that would ensue if all of us who spend our days or nights caring for other people's children took a two-week vacation at the same time:

◀ Manufacturing would grind to a halt.

◀ Wholesale and retail sellers would be unable to open for business.

◀ Hospitals, nursing homes, and clinics would close their doors.

◀ Police stations and fire departments would close.

◀ Elementary and secondary schools would be forced to call a two-week recess.

◀ Spring break would come early for college students and professors alike.

◀ Local, state, and federal government agencies would be incapable of everything from picking up the trash to guarding the nation's borders.

This vision may be slightly exaggerated, but not much. Your profession allows parents to go to work or attend school. If you quit doing your job, they would be unable to do theirs. On top of that, you are providing much-needed early nurturing and educating while parents are away from their children. You are guiding the emotional and physical development of our nation's future. The first woman to visit Mars; a future president; the inventor of the cure for AIDS; the next Mozart, Sinatra, or Bono could be sitting across the room from you eating playdough right now. You are an awesomely important person doing a vital job. A job you probably love . . . or used to.

Rewards and Stressors

And why not love it? Working with children can bring many intangible rewards:

- ◄ Unconditional love from children

- ◄ Heartfelt appreciation from some parents

- ◄ The feeling that you are making a positive difference in the lives of the families you serve

- ◄ Seeing children grow and develop new skills

We get a lot of rewards from this job, but the job also comes with many stressors:

- ◄ Keeping parents happy

- ◄ Assuring children's health and safety

- ◄ Constantly modeling appropriate behavior for kids and good parenting for parents

- ◄ Working long hours that are physically and emotionally demanding

- ◄ Receiving compensation that is often not in line with the demands of the profession

This list could go on for pages, because caregiving is demanding and complex. Research from the Center for the Child Care Workforce shows that every year, 30 to 40 percent of providers drift right out of the profession. This is a disturbing turnover rate, especially when you consider that quality child care is based on strong child/caregiver relationships. The impact such turnover has on children is huge.

The purposes of this book are to offer insight into why caregivers burn out and to provide tools for coping with the stresses that come with your profession. In the following chapters, I will explore who is affected by burnout, why your profession is so prone to it, tools for dealing with burnout, suggestions for handling common stressful situations, and methods to help you get back on the path toward living your Ultimate Purpose. What it boils down to is that the responsibility and stress intrinsic to being an early care and education professional can lead to burnout. I know—it happened to me. I don't want it to happen to you.

Before you read any further, take three or four deep, cleansing breaths and remember that if you're not taking good care of yourself, the care you are providing to others is inadequate too. The only way you can fully be there for those you care for is to fully be there for yourself. I can't offer you any one-size-fits-all answers. There are no easy ways to avoid provider stress and burnout, but if you are willing to do some work, you can make subtle and mindful changes in your life that will put you on a less stressful, more serene path.

Now, take those breaths, relax, and know that you are strong enough to make needed changes in your life.

1

"I Didn't Like You Anymore" — What Burnout Is and How It Changes Your Life

IN MY YEARS AS A PROVIDER, I have cared for children, managed budgets, changed diapers, covered for other staff members, worked through breaks, put in fourteen-hour days, written grants, reported parents for child abuse, hired the wrong people, seen great providers leave the profession, and carried much too much work home in my hands and head. I have provided programming for children ranging in age from infancy to adolescence. I have dealt with parents' problems and problem parents. I've consoled inconsolable infants and, over time, tuned in to their wants and needs. I've spent days on the floor with energetic toddlers, stacking blocks, wiping noses, feeding dolls, receiving hugs lubricated with drool, and rereading the same book over and over again. I've answered preschooler questions until they didn't have another "why" in their heads. I've organized trips to camp, the circus, and the zoo, and I've even planned airplane rides for one hundred school-age children. I've dealt with parents' questions, frustrations, unrealistic expectations, and baseless accusations. I've cried when certain children have left my program, and I've smiled happily to myself when other children have moved on.

I've seen first steps, first words, and first friendships. I've seen tears of gratitude, smiles of appreciation, and looks of admiration. More times than I can count, I've seen that special "ah-ha!" moment when the light of new understanding snaps on over the head of a child. I've experienced all the good and bad that come with being an early care and education professional.

Hundreds of thousands of providers experience these moments on a daily basis as they go about the job of caring for the next generation; you're probably one of those providers.

Along with the good and bad experiences, I have come to know many people from different corners of our profession. I've met great child care professionals and I've met "babysitters" who were anything but professional. Throughout most of my child care career, I have looked at myself as a professional, thought the job was a calling, and believed I was dealing with my stress effectively.

My Story (and Yes—There's a Happy Ending!)

While attending college, I volunteered in a community center after-school program. Over the next four years, my volunteer position turned into a paid job, then into a full-time job, and finally into the community center director's job. After a while, someone suggested that the agency open a child care center and asked me to look into the requirements. Two years later, we opened a child care program in a church basement. Initially, it enrolled one child. After ten years of hard work, that program was housed in a freshly renovated, million-dollar building and served about one hundred children a day. Over that time span, I went from working exclusively with children to working with children *and* computers, files, regulators, administrators, and funders. My main job changed from caregiver to record keeper.

I continued to love the program and my job as its director, but there came a time when I found it increasingly difficult to remember why. The joy that the job once brought me had dwindled, and the workload was constantly increasing. I spent more time reading budgets than *Brown Bear*, more energy explaining the importance of play-based learning to funders than actually playing with children.

I thought everything was okay at the time, but looking back, I can see that I was drifting off course. My mind was shuttled incessantly between yesterday's problems and tomorrow's obligations, and I was veering further away from where I wanted to be: on the floor, blissfully in the moment, playing, exploring, and discovering the world with a group of children.

Still, part of me thought life was going great, right up until the day in early 2003 when I suddenly quit the job I loved, a job I had cherished for over a decade and a half.

It had been a normal day in a normal week until a bit of unwelcome news broke my spirit. It set me off, and I quit a program I had built from nothing. I quit all those kids and their families. I quit something that had become an enormous and ingrained part of my personal identity.

Driving back to the child care center after quitting (my boss's office was at a separate location), I took a good look in the rearview mirror and didn't recognize the person I saw. It was me, but not the me I thought I was, the me I wanted to be. I realized I was burnt out and had been for some time. Deep down, I knew quitting my job was the right thing to do, but I had no idea what came next. Years of repressed stress, frustration, and fear flooded my SUV. Fear, because I was about to tell my beautiful wife, Tasha, what I had just done. You see, for most of my years as a center director, Tasha had been my assistant. She knew that *she* was burning out, and she had wanted to quit her job for years. And all that time, I had been assuring her everything would be okay. I had repeatedly convinced her that things would change, that she would get through it. She had come to me many times and said that she couldn't do it anymore. And I had talked her out of quitting every time. I hadn't seen my own burnout, and I had minimized or ignored hers.

I had to explain to this wonderful, trusting, loving woman that I had just done something I had repeatedly talked her out of doing for at least three years. I cannot fully fathom how shocked she must have been to hear what I had done. She knew better than anyone how much I loved that job and how dedicated I was to it. Explaining my actions to Tasha was one of the most intense and uncomfortable twenty minutes in our marriage. But looking back on it, it was also twenty minutes full of growth, love, connection, and unity—although neither of us uttered those words at the time.

The next morning, Tasha resigned. We both knew that we still wanted to work with children. After a few deep breaths and some thought, we realized that family child care seemed like the path for us to follow. So, in a few months' time, we went from directing a large child care center to being family child care providers. The transition was slow and often tense. Redesigning our lives after total burnout was a challenging task, mentally and emotionally. Years later, I'm still scared to think how close my blind commitment and devotion to a job I loved came to destroying my relationship with my one true love.

I Didn't Like You Anymore

It took a few years, but eventually, and apprehensively, Tasha told me that toward the end of our child care center days, our mutual burnout had reached the point that she no longer liked me. She still loved me, but she no longer enjoyed working with me, and at times didn't even like being around me. Over the course of five or six years, I had gradually become a different person. I had *devolved* into someone she didn't recognize. She didn't like herself for having those feelings, but there they were.

Tasha shared this with me in the spring of 2005—a full two years after we had left the center—while we were driving across Iowa to make a presentation at a conference. I'll never forget it. I had been making notes for this book and had asked for her input when she finally felt comfortable enough to share her feelings. She said, "It had gotten so bad that I didn't like you anymore." I was surprised to hear how strong her feelings were, but they hardly came as a shock. I had been overcommitted to an all-consuming job. We were both putting too much of ourselves into the program, which meant that we were neglecting other parts of our lives—and each other. We worked long hours, and we never left our work behind, even when we left the center.

Back when we were at the center, Tasha wasn't adept at letting me know what was bothering her, and I was generally dismissive when she tried. She, too, had been burning out slowly and steadily for years. Because she had grown up in an environment where she was expected to make the best of bad situations, she had put on a happy face when times grew difficult for her. I could not see behind that happy face, so I was ignorant about her true feelings and to the extent of her burnout. This, combined with ignorance of my *own* feelings, pushed our marriage to the edge of a cliff. If I had not burned out and quit my job, I don't know if we would still be a "we."

It took a long time to put a name to many of the feelings we had struggled with during our burning-out years and even longer for us to feel at ease talking about them with each other. It took quitting our jobs, starting our own family child care program, lots of healing, and a good deal of personal growth before we could comfortably look back and analyze what had happened to us.

I completely understand now why Tasha grew to dislike me. I don't care much for the person I became either. I focused too much on my work and not enough on my family. I became more concerned with the number of children the program served than the individual needs of those children. Over the years, my focus shifted from program quality to program size and finances. There was a long, slow, steady shift in my personal and professional goals. My passion for providing quality early child care and education was slowly replaced by a desire to run a big program in a fancy building. I lost my patience, my direction, my drive, my joy, my passion, and my sense of self. What is scary is that I barely noticed any of those changes until after I quit.

It's difficult for me to share intense feelings with others; like many guys, I tend to internalize my emotions. That may not be the best way to deal with them, but many of us men still hold strong feelings inside until they burst through our chests like the monster in that scene from the movie *Alien*. As uncomfortable as I am sharing my thoughts about burning out, I do it now because I know that I would be even *more* uncomfortable if I didn't.

Spinach

This naturally brings us to spinach.

Not everyone likes spinach, so feel free to substitute another often-stuck-in-the-teeth food for the next few paragraphs. Have you ever had spinach stuck in your teeth and not known about it until some good person was kind enough to tell you? Imagine that you're having dinner, talking, and laughing with friends. After finishing your salad, you try cleaning your teeth unobtrusively with your tongue to avoid the whole spinach-in-the-teeth routine. Unfortunately, one little piece manages to lodge itself next to your upper left canine. You're telling a joke—"This duck and unicorn walk into a bar and order martinis. . . ."—and everyone else is staring at your mouth, specifically at the scrap of spinach flapping with every syllable. But no one says a word to you. You finish the joke. "And the duck says . . ."

Everyone laughs.

An hour later, you overhear a couple talking and chortling: "Did you see him telling that joke?" "I know. I was transfixed by that hunk of spinach in his teeth—it had to be the size of a palm leaf."

Why the heck didn't someone point out the spinach?

Many people are so busy with their own spinach problems that they are oblivious to yours. Others think they might embarrass you or hurt your feelings, so they pretend it isn't there. Some people make discreet gestures to let you know the spinach is there, but you fail to notice. Still others see it and simply don't care enough to tell you. A few folks probably enjoy seeing you walk around with spinach dangling between your teeth. Then there are the brave and blessed few who will look you in the eye and tell you how it is: "You've got spinach between your teeth."

When I think back to my last few years at the center, I realize that many friends and family members had tried to tell me, bravely and directly, that I was on the road to burnout. They could see the spinach, and I could not. I was deaf to their comments and concerns. "You seem tired a lot; how is the job going?" I didn't recognize my burnout until I was ready to. I didn't see the signs. I didn't listen to the people whispering in my ear. I squelched the inner voice that was trying hard to let me know what was up. I knew I had been feeling a bit run down and stressed out as the center's director, but I didn't have any idea how burned out I was until that day when I looked at myself in the rearview mirror, and suddenly, there I was: I saw myself clearly for the first time in years.

The worst our healthy and flavorful friend spinach can do is cause temporary embarrassment. But burnout can mess up or even annihilate your personal and professional relationships, compromise your identity, and impede your ability to reach your goals. Whether you are aware of it or not, burnout makes you lose track of who you are and where you are going. And so it goes. The longer you wander down the path of burnout, the more difficult you'll find it to stop, notice what is going on, and change what you are thinking and doing.

What You Give Is What You Get

In his 2002 book *Meditations from the Mat,* yoga instructor Rolf Gates wrote, "What goes around comes around; whatever we put out into the world comes back onto us." These words could not be truer; it's basic karma. What you give is what you get.

The people in our lives deserve better than we are able to give them when we are experiencing burnout. It blinds us, weakens us, and diminishes our abilities. If you're a provider who is experiencing burnout, you are not a provider on top of your game. Burnout is your kryptonite, draining your power to tune in to your own needs and those of the people you care for. When you're burning out, you are offering the world an inferior product, and that is what comes back to you.

I almost let burnout destroy my marriage. I love walking up behind

Tasha during the day, grasping her slender waist and kissing the back of her neck. I look forward to falling asleep with her each night, and I dream of waking next to her each morning. I love the two beautiful babies we made together. I love her patience with me, her tolerance of my whims, her lovingness, her kindheartedness, her generosity. She is the most important person in my life. I hope to never again allow myself to forget that I was once so burned out that Tasha no longer liked me.

I can spot a burned-out child care provider from across a crowded room at a conference by the way she carries herself and interacts with her environment. I can look in her eyes and see that she is stressed, run down, and empty. Burnout hardly ever shows up without its best buddy, stress, but feeling stressed doesn't necessarily mean you're burned out. We all feel stress at times, but people who are burning out describe feeling stressed and out of gas on a regular basis, and this means that they've let stress accumulate over a period of time. Too many of us live lives that are not equipped with operable release valves; we have no healthy ways of discharging pressure. One way or another, that pressure must get released. It could happen as it did with me—all at once, in a big bang. More likely, it will happen as it did with Tasha, slowly over time, with a whimper.

How Child Care Providers Are Like Lightbulbs

Providers are prone to burnout because we deal so closely with the emotions of other people and because our job requires us to be sustainedly empathetic. Living inside the heads of the children we care for is part of our job. We need to tune in to their emotional needs as part of getting to know them well, and we need to know them well to meet their needs successfully. This emotional closeness is something most of us love about the job, but it is also a big contributor to burnout. At times it becomes hard to separate ourselves from those we care for, to detach from their lives and to focus on our own.

The term *burnout* was probably imported from the field of electrical engineering. When electrical components are forced to handle too much current, they overheat and burn out. A burned-out lightbulb is no longer part of the electrical circuit to which it is connected. This means energy can no longer flow freely to and from the bulb; the filament is fried, so the bulb no longer gives off light. An electrical motor that receives too much current spins and spins, generating lots of heat, until it finally fails. It's the same with people. We burn out, and our light dims; our motors seize, and our energy stops flowing. We disconnect from the people who are dear to us. Jobs once viewed as hallowed turn dark and difficult. We drift, losing sight of our life's dreams, goals, and direction.

Let me offer you another metaphor: In drag racing, drivers intentionally induce a burnout of their tires before their runs in order to generate heat and improve friction. They spin their tires in place, generating plumes of smoke and lots of heat and friction. This is great if you're a drag racer, but all the smoke, heat, and friction generated by a caregiver's burnout is damaging. I've seen providers busily spinning their tires, quickly going nowhere, and generating lots of heat from the friction in their lives. All the while, they keep blowing smoke about how well they are doing.

I have vowed never to allow burnout to take over my life again, but I also know I am not immune to it. Every word of this book was written before or after long days with a group of great kids, during naptime, or during my much-too-short weekends. There have been times when managing my family obligations, my job as a provider, this book, and the rest of my life became stressful. I still enjoy taking on new challenges and working up to my own high expectations. The difference is that now I've made changes in my life that allow me to deal directly with my stress, vent my frustrations openly, and meet my own needs. I'm always looking in the mirror for burnout (and spinach).

In the next chapter, I will look at who is affected by burnout and describe the damage. In the chapters that follow, I will examine why child care professionals are so prone to burnout and how to make changes in your life that will help you avoid it. If you're already a victim of burnout, I'll describe techniques for healing the damage you've already done.

REFERENCE

Gates, Rolf, and Katrina Kenison. 2002. *Meditations from the Mat: Daily Reflections on the Path of Yoga*. New York: Anchor Books.

Time Out

Twenty Minutes in the Life of...

Child care is hard work. See if you can relate to anything in the following scenario:

It's 9:37 on Monday morning, and you're in a child care center room with ten three-year-olds—two over your state's limit for this age group. It's just an average Monday, but you've been dreading it since Sunday morning. You're only seven minutes into the workday, and it feels like a long week already. You're tired and bored, your neck and back hurt, you're out of patience and easily upset, and you're fed up with being fed up. It's probably not the kids who are responsible for your mood, although they may have helped. You love them all. The one whose nose has been constantly running since you met her over two years ago gives such affectionate hugs. The quicker-than-lightning biter who loves books and is such a joy during story time. The boy who, at age three and a half, still has no interest in potty training and is so curious and eager to discover new things. The anything-but-perfect twins with the overly concerned, perfectionist mother. You look at the snot, the biting, and all the rest as challenges that you can help them deal with, maybe even overcome. You're good at it, too; that is why you have put up with so much for so long. You love to see the children grow, explore the world, and reach new milestones. The problem is that the road bumps in your day have turned into mountains, and this has been the case for quite some time. You just do not have the patience and energy to deal with these issues as well as you would like. You catch yourself being short with the children, their parents, your coworkers, your own family; even the dog now feels your wrath.

As you attempt to warm up to the day, parents run in, drop off kids, and run out. When they stop to chat, it is usually to complain; a simple *thank you* would be so nice to hear now and then. You assume that they appreciate you, but hearing the words spoken would do a lot for your morale. It's just you and the kids until eleven o'clock. The isolation that comes with this job is sometimes too much to take. You are preoccupied, hoping that the new part-time girl makes it to work so you can get at least one break today. You would be watching the parking lot to see if she pulls in, but you're in a windowless room. She's a sophomore at the local college and seems nice enough, but she has missed five Mondays in the six weeks since she was hired. She claims she was sick. "How lucky for her," you think sarcastically. "I could use a few three-day weekends before she quits or gets fired. Turnover is so high around here that I'll never get my vacation." You'd like to complain, but the director seems to be ducking you—she looks as stressed out as you feel.

You get to work on time and do your job and wish everyone else would do the same. All you seem to get for being dependable is un-wanted extra hours and missed breaks. You always end up picking up the slack for someone else.

9:40. The heavy clouds finally burst with rain. It's a nice, gentle, warm rain, and the kids would enjoy playing outside while it is falling. Outside time in the rain would be a wonderful sensory activity, but the fact is you just don't have the energy to get all of them ready to go out and then deal with the wet mess afterward. Soaked socks, shoes, and clothes: nothing would dry before naptime, and some parents would probably complain about the wetness. You feel a bit guilty for not putting in the effort, but you just don't have the energy. You'll just stay inside—it's simpler, less stressful. It's going to be a long and loud day. The kids have been away since Friday, and over the weekend all of them have forgotten how to behave. They always seem extra tired, rude, grumpy, and foul on Monday morning.

You had believed that it was only the kids in *your* program that were like this until you went to an organizational meeting for a local providers' support group. You had a great conversation with a few other providers and heard that their kids acted just like yours in many ways. It was nice to share concerns and vent to the other providers who attended; you had so much in common with them. The goal of the meeting had been to create a group that would meet monthly for training and for discussing child care issues. It was a good idea, but who has the time or energy to meet after a full day's work? It was a fun get-together, but you haven't made it to any more meetings and probably won't. After work these days, you just want to go home and veg out in front of the TV.

9:48. Simone is biting again, and Taylor has wet his pants. You try to give the kids the individual attention they need to help them through these phases, but your time is stretched so thin and your patience is at the breaking point. Sometimes you just want to scream. That pain in your neck always seems to flair up at work—it doesn't bother you nearly as much on the weekends. You know it's stress related, but what can you do about it? You have to work, so you have to deal with the stress that comes with the job. You do want to deal with it more effectively. You realize that sitting on the couch every night and shopping too much every weekend doesn't seem to be doing the trick. Making changes would be good, but it would also require some physical effort on your part. The thought of doing anything is exhausting; you feel you're just not ready for the effort.

9:56. You cringe as your wisdom tooth flares up again. You need to get it fixed, but it's going to cost more than you have in your savings account. You try not to think about it, but it sure can't be ignored much longer. Having a job with insurance would be great.

9:58. You're tired, tense, anxious, stiff, stressed out, pissed off, and it's not even ten o'clock. Sadly, this is what you have come to think of as a normal day—even a *good* day.

2

Who Burnout Hurts and What the Hurt Looks Like

WHEN I DO PRESENTATIONS on burnout in workshops around the country, I hear a lot of personal stories from providers who are in various stages of recognizing and dealing with the stress and challenges of working in this profession. While there are common themes running through most of their stories, each one reflects the unique way in which each of us experiences burnout.

Two Providers, Two Different Burnout Stories

The following is from an e-mail I received from a center provider who attended one of my presentations:

> I can feel I'm not doing the job I used to do. It's just not in me anymore. I don't feel I'm doing what I was meant to do. I often think of what I have not done with my life and the things I want to do. The center is not what it used to be, or maybe I'm not what I used to be. I feel that I've worked there ten years and have gotten nowhere. No opportunity for advancement or better pay. I don't feel a part of it.
>
> It would be easy to blame the directors, the staff, coworkers, or parents. The big problem is me. I have choices and I need to take responsibility for my choices. I took the job, I stayed at the job. You

*have to give up complaining and work to make things better or
get out. You can't do a good job feeling resentments. When you
know it's time to get out, go. Trust your gut. Sometimes it gets to
a point where there's nothing that would help with your burnout
except another job in another career. If you stay, you're doing no
one any good.*

A year later, I checked in to see if this provider had made any
changes. She was still working at the same center in the same position. She said, "Things have changed somewhat since I started being
more assertive and simply not taking crap anymore. The thing that
keeps me there is [that] the parents and children like me, that means
I'm doing my job well; that's who I'm there for in the first place." She
has worked hard for a long time at a job about which she says, "I'm
not doing the job I used to do. It's just not in me anymore." She stays
because she feels she is meeting the needs of the parents and children.
She's burned out but hanging on because she thinks she is doing
something good for someone else. She's not alone in her feelings
or her rationale for sticking with a job she no longer loves or loves
equivocally.

Notice the similarities and the difference between the woman I
quoted above and the following words of a family child care provider,
who shared her thoughts with me on another occasion:

*Most of why I went through such burnout is due to a great deal of
stress and frustration. Most of the stress has been due to my husband and me struggling with an infertility issue. I've been taking
care of these children for so long, and I put in all I've got, and I
started to feel like I was pretty much raising them but yet they still
weren't "mine." That was really hard, especially because I develop a
genuine love for the kids in my care. So, at the bottom of the "little"
things that bugged me, was this huge painful issue.*

*Finances also played a large part in my almost quitting. My hus-
band has a job that he loves, but it sure doesn't pay a doctor's salary!
I also love my job, but we all know child care providers are paid far
less than they're worth. So, finances seem constantly strained for*

us. I was having trouble affording what I needed for the child care week plus what we needed for ourselves. Also, two families left me, one of which gave no notice and refused to return or answer my phone calls. That wreaked havoc with my self-esteem and made me imagine all sorts of horrible reasons why they would do that to me.

It got to the point that I just carried this constant stress around with me, making me over[re]act when the kids would misbehave, and leaving me feeling like a terrible person who shouldn't be caring for children at all. So, guilt came into play as well. I was constantly stressed out and feeling horrible guilt for not being "perfect." I've always struggled with being a perfectionist, and I felt I could never meet my own standards. It was very self-defeating.

Notice that in her analysis of her situation, this provider was aware that her dissatisfaction was not *all* tied to her child care work; she had important personal issues (infertility and guilt) that she acknowledged and needed to explore. Ultimately, this provider dealt with the issues that drove her from her career as a caregiver and worked to get things back on track personally and professionally. She took action on both the financial and personal fronts to make her life happier and her career more viable and stable. She raised her rates (and was shocked when families agreed without hesitation to her higher fees), and she and her husband began to look into possibly adopting. "That decision alone took an enormous amount of stress out of my life," she said.

Life Is Messy, and Then Some

Going to the effort to find, buy, and read this book means you probably have at least a nodding relationship with burnout. If the details in the stories above are not yours, you can certainly relate to some of the feelings of these two providers. Life, whether you are a caregiver or not, can become stressful, frustrating, and downright messy. Working in a caring profession like counseling, nursing, and child care can only compound such problems.

You need to acknowledge that as a child care provider, you often struggle with not only the normal challenges of living but with others unique to caregivers, like the ones I've quoted above: low wages; demanding workload; and uncommonly complex, intense relationships. An April 2001 report from the Wilder Research Center showed that 42 percent of family child care providers left the profession annually because of burnout. The same report indicated that providers from center- and home-based programs, as well as Head Start, preschool, and school-age programs, identified the following as contributions to their decision to leave the profession:

◀ dissatisfaction with wages

◀ disappointment with benefits

◀ job stress

◀ conflict with coworkers or supervisors

◀ need to socialize with other adults

◀ desire to work shorter hours

All of these motivations for abandoning the profession of early care and education are major contributors to provider burnout. Admittedly, many providers who leave the field, burned out or not, are simply not suited to the profession. But many more experienced, dedicated, and educated caregivers walk away from jobs they love because they can no longer handle the strain. Their departure negatively affects the morale of those left behind, who must struggle to fill the void.

This regular loss of experienced providers is detrimental to children, families, and communities. Margaret K. Nelson, in her 1990 report "A Study of Turnover among Family Day Care Providers," stated, "The child care literature today is rife with reports about high rates of burnout and turnover among child care workers. These phenomena can have a devastating impact on children who are thereby deprived of enthusiastic and continuous care." Even worse than the burnout problem is the fact that so many years after her study, the topic is not more researched or discussed.

Providers who are burned out and remain in the profession without effectively dealing with the problem have a huge negative impact on the quality of care that children receive. Providers who have lost their enthusiasm but who stay on because they feel they have no other choice are much less likely to provide children with the close, nurturing, loving, individualized care they need and deserve. Too many child care programs in this country have staff who, because of burnout, are little more than warm bodies present to make sure the program adheres to mandated staff-to-child ratios.

In the book *Finding a Path with a Heart: How to Go from Burnout to Bliss,* Beverly Potter defined burnout as "a loss of enthusiasm, a surrendering of ambition, a sense of resignation that consumes the spirit and can even lead to physical ailments. Burnout is a stressful process accompanied by declining performance, people problems, feelings of meaninglessness, negative emotions, frequent illness, and a propensity to engage in substance abuse." If this describes you as a provider, you are not in a position to help the children in your care shine brightly. You cannot tune in to their needs and desires when you yourself are out of tune.

Most providers are familiar with at least a few of the stressors that I've mentioned so far. As caregivers, we often work in environments that are not conducive to our mental well-being—environments that are physically and emotionally stressful, environments that leave us feeling used and abused.

A clearer understanding of what you are up against can help you clarify your thinking and make it easier to chart a healthier relationship with yourself. So before I look at ways to survive, overcome, and avoid the devastation that burnout causes, I'm going to look closely at the reasons so many caregivers fizzle out and leave the profession in the first place and the impact that burnout has on them and those around them.

Burnout and Relationships

Burnout messes up interpersonal connections. My burnout drove me to a place where I trampled on people important to me, berated near strangers, and ignored people who needed my attention. No one has ever shared an anecdote about how sneaky tooth-spinach almost destroyed her marriage or made her leave a job, but I hear about burnout doing these things all the time. The profession of early care and education is about building and maintaining strong, true, sacred, and honest relationships. When you burn out, you change. You cheat your family and friends, coworkers, peers, the children you care for, and yourself. You fail to focus fully on what's important. Burnout blinds you to the importance of interpersonal dealings and obscures previously open relationships. It leads you away from the people in your life. Your sightless eyes miss the interplay in social-emotional dealings with other people, and you become unable to participate fully in the present moments. This is tragic, since the best times in life are spent intimately with others in the sacred now.

Let's examine the key relationships that burnout can sabotage:

◀ Family and friends

◀ Coworkers and peers

◀ Children in your care

◀ Your identity

◀ Your goals

Family and Friends

Child care is a hard profession to leave at the workplace. You may leave work, but most providers I've talked to report that work very rarely leaves them. It's always there in a corner of your conscious mind. You worry about the kids, fret about the budget, second-guess your decisions and actions, and repeatedly replay events in your head. The job consumes you. No matter how much you try, separating work from family seems nearly impossible. The job follows most providers home at the end of the day. And those of you who are family providers have it even worse; work happens right there in your home. The strong emotions, good and bad; the daily highlights and lowlights; the stress and anxiety; the psychological ups and downs; and the physical strain are all likely to find their way into your family life.

I've talked to many providers who would like to go home and vent about job-related stress to their significant others but have a hard time doing so because their spouses are uninterested, belittling, too busy, or otherwise unwilling to listen. Their spouses don't understand (or don't *want* to understand) the profession enough to be of any help, or worse, they dismiss the problems as inconsequential. My personal experience is that providers would simply like to go home and have someone listen—not comment, not make jokes, not try to solve problems, not make suggestions—just listen.

The problem is that many spouses and children are stressed out from their own days. They may feel the need to blow off steam themselves, so they aren't available to listen to your problems. They may deflect the issue by joking around and passing your problems off as not so serious. Many just aren't interested in anything related to child care; they simply won't talk about it or they'll listen impatiently while thinking about something they consider more important. What is sometimes even worse, they may try to help by offering logical, pat solutions and avoiding discussion of the most important part: your feelings.

Humans are social creatures, and it is often difficult just to sit and listen. You want to share your opinions and comments, solve problems, and carry on discussions. Sitting quietly is hard to do; allowing someone to let out his feelings is even harder. The situation is even more complicated when the person you want to share work-related feelings and experiences with is unwilling to listen. This often leads to conflict in the relationship that will either escalate into other problems or choke off communication about what's happening at work altogether. Neither option is productive or healthy for the people in your household.

When Tasha and I were both burning out, we got to the point where we would come home and almost ignore each other much of the time. Because I was blind to my own burnout, I held her responsible for our lack of communication, and I wouldn't accept my share of the blame. When she did try to talk to me about what was bugging her, I would try to solve the problems. I wanted to fix things for her. She wanted me to shut up and listen.

Things are much better now. I've learned how to shut up and just listen, and Tasha has learned to talk about problems before they reach a boiling point. Through our experience of burnout, we have both learned to communicate more effectively. We now have less to feel stressed about, and we have both learned to handle our stress more successfully.

Coworkers and Peers

Leaving my position as a center director meant leaving a group of people who had become family. When you spend each workday, week after week, year after year, with a particular group of people, you develop close relationships. If you work in a school or center and have coworkers, think about how much you share with them: birthdays, marriages, divorces, births, deaths, smiles, tears—life! When you find yourself neglecting these relationships, this may be a sign of burnout. Looking back, I can see how burnout caused me to hurt my relationships with coworkers:

- ◢ I looked for opportunities to pull rank. I started giving orders and laying down the law instead of empowering my staff. It was easier to be The Boss than to be A Leader.

- ◢ I rushed decision making. I chose quick decision making over mindful contemplation and informed decision making so I could swiftly move to the next item on my too-full agenda. I began to focus more on the product than the process. This, of course, often led to bad decisions and upset staff.

- ◢ I became a rigid, by-the-book kind of guy. I lost the flexibility I once had with staff members who were dealing with difficult situations in their personal lives.

- ◢ I isolated myself. I was so stressed that it was a relief to hide in my office with the door closed. I took every opportunity to be away from the center. It was easier to leave for a meeting than to deal with the staff and kids. (This meant more work, pressure, and stress for Tasha, my wife and assistant.)

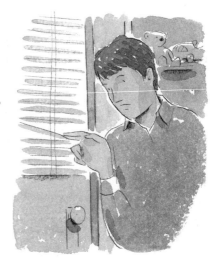

◄ I lost my patience. I got to the point where I couldn't tolerate . . . well, anything!

These and other changes in my personality tore me away from coworkers. They were pieces of a wall I unconsciously built around myself. The same process was occurring among my peers. Once a month for a number of years while I was a center director, I would get together with a group of four or five other directors. We would meet for a late lunch and vent. We discussed a variety of issues related to staffing, parents, kids, regulators, and funding. We talked about how to solve the world's problems. This regular get-together became an oasis for us each month, a small island of opportunity to let off steam safely in understanding company. We discussed many important things, but the conversation always turned eventually to frustrations, troubles, stresses—and burnout. Looking back, I recognize that I perversely started to pull away from this group as my burnout intensified. I tried to isolate myself from the very people who understood my state of mind better than anyone else. I don't know if I was afraid that they would see through the wall I was building to protect myself or if I was frightened because I was starting to see myself in their stories.

Children in Your Care

I've thought often about a certain child Tasha and I cared for in our family care setting. She had not been dealt the best hand in life.

Leaving our program after spending much of her first eighteen months with us was just one of many upheavals she experienced in her tumultuous young life. Many providers care for children in similar situations. There are too many children with broken families, struggling parents, chaotic home lives, and messy personal histories. Too often, children are treated as fashion accessories, punching bags, personal burdens, playthings, or drains on family resources. Sometimes parents with good intentions do not have the skills, resources, or aptitude to care well for their children. In all of these cases, the children suffer. Such children are often desperate for the structure, warmth, safety, dependability, openness, serenity, and unconditional love they might receive in your child care program. Your house or center becomes the safe port in whatever storm they are weathering. These storm-tossed children are seldom easy to care for. Their turbulent young lives have left battle scars, behavioral problems, and annoying idiosyncrasies that make emotional closeness difficult for them and you.

Difficult, but not impossible. These children require extra effort on your part. You have to grit your teeth to get past the obstacles they have constructed for their own protection. Tuning in to the special needs of these children is a huge challenge. You need to build emotional bridges to them and gently break down the walls they have built around their hearts. As a caregiver, you give of yourself. You make connections happen. You get close.

Getting in step with any child can be difficult; you have to dedicate yourself to the goal of being fully there for them in all dealings at all times, even when you know you won't always be able to meet it. I know this is a lofty and almost impossible-sounding goal. It's not easy, but few things are in the child care profession. The children sometimes crawl right under your skin. They irritate you easily but unintentionally. You find yourself feeling frustrated and mad at them for all kinds of reasons: spilt milk, runny noses, tantrums, inconsiderate parents—insert your pet peeve here. It can be a struggle to get past these challenges to what is really important: building a strong and solid bond with children so you can better meet their needs.

Such feelings of anger and frustration are far from unique or rare, but they are often difficult to admit. You want to think (and to have others believe) that you're beyond such thoughts. However, what you really have to do is face the fact that having these feelings is perfectly natural, and then you can move beyond them so that you're fully present for the children in your care. Mimi Brodsky Chenfeld, author of *Celebrating Young Children and Their Teachers*, described the time providers spend engaged with children as "sacred interactions" in her keynote address to the 2006 South Dakota Association for the Education of Young Children conference. *Sacred Interactions:* blessed, holy, spiritual, divine, deep, meaningful, profound, important, celestial, significant interactions. These daily exchanges with children are so important and yet are often so difficult to be fully present for. Mimi's words reminded me that my burnout took away the joy of such interactions, which I had valued deeply. Trapped behind the wall I was building to protect myself from burnout, I was unable to reach out to the kids.

I started working in this profession because I enjoyed the magical moments when I was able to help things "click" for children. Such interactions faded away as I began spending most of my time staring at a computer or going to meetings instead of playing dodgeball, reading *Good Families Don't*, stacking blocks, digging in the sand, or just hanging out with the kids. I had allowed the piece of the job I valued most to slip away. It saddens me to think about the sacred moments I missed because I allowed burnout to wrap me up in myself.

Refreshed and renewed, I now start each day focused on play instead of payroll, relationships instead of reports, discovery instead of day planners. I'll be sitting on the floor observing my one-year-old friend Sam happily at play with cute little Kia or his two-year-old cousin, Ty. Looking across the room with a gleam in his eye, Sam steamrolls toward me. *CRASH!* I fall backward, and he sits straddling my chest, all smiles and drool, eyes still shining. Our eyes lock. Then it starts. His right index finger slides skillfully into my left ear. I quiver and shake. He laughs and babbles. Again the finger goes in the ear and I shake . . . and again . . . and again. He laughs gleefully each time his finger creeps toward my ear. I shake and shudder on cue as soon as there is contact. After five, ten, maybe fifty cycles of the finger-in-the-ear game, he puts his cheek to mine and gives me a hug.

The responsibilities that tore me away from kids before my burnout are still there, but I no longer allow them to take over my life. Child care is all about relationships, about being not only physically but emotionally and spiritually present for children. Relationships like the one I have with Sam are the most important part of our profession, and anything that hurts those relationships is dangerous. Being fully there is often hard, even when your life is full of sunshine, cotton candy, and daisies, and nearly impossible when you are burning out.

Stressed caregivers influence children in another way: what kids see is what they learn. Their keen eyes are always on you, reading your body language, sharing your stress, feeding on your energy. Children in the care of an adult who is centered, calm, and comfortable in her own skin are usually happy and contented children. Children with a frazzled caregiver feed off his negative energy and act accordingly. Imagine a stressed provider surrounded by five or six fussing, fighting, fidgeting, and unfocused children. The provider has a headache; the kids are bouncing off the walls. The provider is preoccupied with her thoughts; the kids are one-upping each other in their bid to gain her attention. The provider is irritable; the kids don't know how to behave because they are getting mixed signals.

Is the provider stressed because of the children's behavior, or are the children acting this way because of the provider's stress? I once had a chance to chat with Michelle, a dedicated provider in Missouri, during lunch at a conference. We sat outside in the warm spring sun, eating our boxed lunches, while she shared an experience from the center where she works. The director had fired the girl Michelle worked with for falling asleep on the job. The girl had been missing work a lot and had not been the best employee. The children responded to the vibe she was putting out—they were undomesticated beasts when she was in charge. The dismissal meant that, until a replacement could be hired, the remaining staff had to cover her hours. The children had to be shuffled from room to room, forced to spend time in the care of providers they did not know, and confused about the sudden absence of the terminated employee. All these changes in their routine stressed the children even more. They acted out, fought, bit, fussed, and generally misbehaved. It took a while to hire a replacement and even longer for the children to become comfortable with the new caregiver and for the program to reassume normalcy.

When you allow yourself to get run down, stressed out, anxious, overly tired, and empty, how can you expect to give the kind of care that children need and deserve? If you are running on empty, how can you expect to fuel them with a passion for life and learning? If you are stressed, how can you provide them with a calm and relaxed environ-ment? If you are experiencing your own inner storms, how can you expect to calm theirs? If you are burned out, how can you keep your interactions sacred?

Children deserve better than that; they deserve providers who are fully focused and happy at their work.

Your Identity

Burnout can become so bad that it becomes part of who you are. It snakes its way into your life and personality, enveloping you. Instead of remaining Husband, Wife, Teacher, Caregiver, Mom, Dad, Friend, Coworker, or Neighbor, you become your burnout. In turn, others perceive you through the lens of your burnout. Burnout changes you in a steady, slow, and subtle manner. Over time, happy, outgoing, en-ergetic, vibrant people become depressed, reclusive, unmotivated, and apathetic. I personally had to hit rock-bottom before I noticed these changes in myself. While you are burning out, you may fail to see what is happening, because people tend to look at themselves through protective lenses and filters. On some level, it is easier not to see the problem than to address it.

When I finally looked in that rearview mirror after quitting my job, I was able to see how my identity had shifted. I was no longer the same person, and I was scared. I didn't want to be the person I had become, but at that moment, I did not know how to be anyone else.

I set to work reconnecting with myself, rebuilding my identity. For about six months after leaving my center job, I cut myself off from my prior world and most of the people I had worked with. It took time and work, but I finally reached the point where I was happy with the person I saw in the mirror. I used most of the techniques that I describe in chapter 4 and reestablished *me*. The most interesting element to me is that when I finally started bringing the people I had distanced myself from back into my life, many said thinks like, "You look different!" "What did you change?" "You look younger!" and "Did you lose weight or change your hair?" Not only had burnout altered my inner identity—it had also changed the way I looked. Once I had refreshed myself spiritually and emotionally, my physical appearance changed too. Now, when I walk though the halls at a conference or other gathering of providers, I see how I must have looked reflected in other people who have burned out; I can spot it in the way they carry themselves. I see burnout weighing them down, compressing their bodies. It is almost as if the emotional and spiritual pressure they are under physically constricts them: their brows furrow, their faces tighten, their shoulders pull forward and up, their necks shrink into their torsos, their torsos sink into their hips, their arms draw in to their sides, and their gait shortens. Like me at my worst, they are so burned out that even their physical appearance and identity have changed. If you allow it to, burnout will slowly and relentlessly change you, inside and out.

Your Goals

Like your relationships and personal identity, burnout influences your goals by insidiously shifting your focus. One day you have a clear set of personal and professional goals that you are working toward making a reality, and then, seemingly in the blink of an eye, you're drifting aimlessly or, worse yet, running aground and stagnating. Burnout immobilizes you. It shreds your dreams, desires, and aspirations if you let it.

I know providers who have given up their aspirations to write, hang glide, dance, rock climb, find true love, lose weight, travel, learn to play an instrument, or walk the Appalachian Trail because they no longer feel they are able to. They have relinquished hope for change. Even if you can remember your dreams, you'll find it hard to work to achieve them when burnout is blurring your vision. Your mind becomes hazy, and you lose your ability to make good decisions amid the fog. During my own burnout, I felt as if I were moving through thick, oozy oatmeal. For a while, I had a vague recollection of what my goals had been, but I was so busy fighting the oatmeal that I was unable to focus on where I wanted to go. Finally, day-to-day life became so busy and complicated that my dreams simply faded into the distance. They slowly started to reappear on the horizon once I began working to recover from my burnout. But it took time and effort to get back on track. In chapter 6, I'll talk about how to set goals so that you can make your dreams a reality and achieve your Ultimate Purpose.

I've painted a grim picture, but there's a bright side to it: if you can begin to move through life more mindfully from moment to moment, you can change habits and routines, alter your thinking, and make room for activities that refresh your mind and body. You do not have to lose your cherished connections with family members, friends, children, and dreams. If you feel that those connections have already been lost, know that you can probably rekindle them if you are willing to make the effort. Before discussing ways to counteract burnout in chapter 4, I am going to examine why providers are so susceptible to it in the first place. Then I'll look at tools you can use to reverse the effects of burnout so that you can banish it from your life.

REFERENCES

Chase, Richard A. 2001. "Staff Recruitment and Retention in Early Childhood Care and Education and School-Age Care." Wilder Research Center. www.wilder.org/fileadmin/user_upload/research/staffing4-01.pdf.

Nelson, Margaret K. 1990. "A Study of Turnover among Family Day Care Providers." *Children Today* 19, no. 2.

Potter, Beverly. 1994. *Finding a Path with a Heart: How to Go from Burnout to Bliss*. Berkeley, Calif.: Ronin Books.

Time Out

Some Tips for Those of You Who Don't Have Enough Stress in Your Life

Burnout and stress may be as foreign to you as traditional Uzbekistani folk dancing. You may be the calmest and coolest person in any room you enter. You may actually be looking for ways to add stress to your life so that you can understand what the rest of us are fussing about. If so, here are some tips.

How to Add Stress to Your Life

▲ Help each child in your care lose a sock or shoe every day for two weeks. When parents ask what's going on, just shrug and smile.

▲ Enact a no-nap policy.

▲ Every time a parent makes a request, smile, say, "I'll take care of it," and completely forget the request as soon as possible. Never mention it again. If the parent brings it up, act confused and puzzled.

▲ Forget ratios—the more, the merrier!

▲ Three words: toddlers, scissors, kittens.

▲ Work longer hours and burn 25 percent of your income each payday.

▲ Avoid trying anything new. Any excuse will do: *It's too messy. It's too expensive. There's not enough time. The kids won't like it.* This ensures hours of whiny, bored youngsters and the stress that they bring.

◄ Tell everyone you meet what you think about everything . . . all the time. Give advice freely, especially on topics you know nothing about. The stress you add to the lives of others will come back to you threefold.

◄ Add at least three items to your to-do list for each task you complete.

◄ Be a minimum of forty minutes late everywhere you go.

◄ Play loud music for the children all day, every day.

◄ Expect perfection from everyone you come into contact with: the children, the parents, your family, and *especially* yourself!

◄ Don't let emotional wounds heal—pick away the scab every chance you get. Adopt a "Let It Fester" policy.

◄ Cut communication with parents in your program (and your loved ones) down to once a week. Talk less and grunt more. If there are problems or concerns, hold off even longer.

◄ Swear off outdoor time for the kids. Make any excuse for keeping them indoors every day. Then act surprised when the yelling, running, and fighting start.

◄ Quit sleeping, give up exercise, and eat anything you want.

◄ Make time with your significant other every day to doubt, shout, and pout.

◄ Stop accepting payment for care. Just do it because you love it so much.

◄ Ignore inquisitive four-year-olds.

▲ Let the phone ring twenty times before answering. If it's a parent, pretend you get disconnected. Keep the ringer set as loud as possible, especially during quiet time.

▲ Forget nutritional guidelines. Serve only sugary food, Kool-Aid, cookies, and the Halloween candy you stock up on each year when it goes on clearance.

▲ Buy eleven blue chairs and one pink chair for the pre-schoolers to use.

This list was compiled with the help of providers via the Family Child Care Professionals of South Dakota Web site, www.sdfcc.org.

3

"I Can't Smile at the Kids Anymore"—Signs of Burnout

THE TITLE OF THIS CHAPTER is the answer a provider gave when asked, during a conference session on burnout, "How do you know when you're burning out?" The respondent was the lead teacher in a preschool room who had worked with young children for over twenty years. She responded, "I know it's getting to me when I can't smile at the kids anymore. I don't take joy in the silly little things they do throughout the day like I used to. I don't have the energy to be happy." Her words were met by a sea of heads nodding knowingly. You will probably recognize other responses to this question that have resonated with providers:

- "The little things get to me, like lost socks and runny noses. Things that are just part of the job stress me out."

- "I'm tired all the time and can't get enough sleep."

- "I just about lose it with the kids because I find myself tying the same shoe over and over again. It's not their fault and it's no big deal—it just gets under my skin."

- "I know I'm feeling burned out when I can't seem to get to work on time. I don't intend to be late, but I'm just not motivated like I used to be. It comes in cycles. Sometimes

I'll be feeling great, and other times I'm dragging for weeks at a time."

It's Your Environment—*and* It's You

Many of us have a tendency to blame somebody else for everything that goes wrong in our lives. If we run out of milk at lunchtime, it's the cook's fault; if the kids are loud, it's the assistant's fault for getting them all riled up; if it rains on a trip to the zoo, it's the weatherman's fault. But when we start experiencing symptoms of burnout like the ones I listed from the providers at my workshops, then we often start blaming ourselves. The causes of burnout are rarely as simple as all-me or all-somebody-else. The truth is, burnout is usually caused by a mix of the environment you work in and the choices you make about how you relate to that environment. For child care providers in particular, environment is often the bigger player. Still, your actions and reactions play a large part in determining how your environment—the people, places, and things that you interact with every day—affects you. You can't always control your work conditions and environment, but you do have a lot of control over how you respond to them.

Burnout guru Christina Maslach addressed situational stress in her book *Burnout: The Cost of Caring*, asserting that it is caused by the environment within which you interact. Maslach pointed out that, like police officers, therapists, and social workers, child care providers work in environments that are conducive to emotional overload. These environments call for too much emotional involvement, too much work, and too much responsibility, all of which result in too much pressure. If you haven't developed the right self-awareness and coping skills, those stressors, coupled with lack of time off, appreciation, resources, and breathing space, build up until BOOM!—your system overloads, and you burn out. You blame yourself—"If I was better at this job, I could keep four infants happy all day long"—and others—"If *they* would provide better supplies and a pay increase, I could really do more for these preschoolers." In reality, you choose your responses to the stressful, exhausting surrounding you work in. It is these choices, along with the environmental factors themselves, that can lead to burnout—or to reducing stress and keeping your smile.

A Toxic Environment

After leaving my job as center director, I held myself responsible for not having been able to handle the job. I felt that I had not been up to the task. This depressed me. Fortunately, over time, I came to realize that although I could have made better choices, the main problem had been my work environment. This hunch was confirmed when nearly ten of my coworkers left the organization within a year after I quit. Even more people would have left if they had felt they could afford the financial and emotional uncertainty. An agency that had once offered meaningful, emotionally rewarding, and enjoyable work had become a breeding ground for insecurity, anxiety, and stress.

This was a tragedy for the people who left the organization, and it was also tragic for the community. As more skilled, dedicated employees burned out and left the agency, volunteers began to jump ship too, and programs began to close. First, a meal program that served low-income children shut down, then the community center that was a safe haven for those children, then basketball and volleyball programs serving hundreds of girls in the community, and finally the child care center itself. The environment had become so toxic that the place imploded.

Saying that caregivers get attached to their programs only states the obvious; your program becomes part of you. I still sometimes wonder: If I had done things differently, would those closed programs still be around? If I had handled my burnout better, could I have soldiered through? Did I fail the children by leaving?

The man who had hired me left the agency a few months after I did. He had soldiered on until he could no longer take it. Paul "Sonny" Kellen was four years old when he walked into the community center he would one day direct; the place was part of his daily life for more than forty years. We were coworkers for over a decade and a half, and some weeks we spent more time together at work than we did at home with our wives. He hired me, he mentored me, he taught me that the workplace could be a place with heart, and he showed me that every situation could be handled with a smile. Unhappily, I learned how to burn out from him too. I saw that he fully submerged himself in his job, and I did the same. I saw how his devotion to the center was straining his marriage, but I didn't notice what it was doing to mine. I saw it affecting his health, but I did not see that it was hurting mine. In the end, we both burned out, and we both emerged from the ashes happier and healthier.

The Signs of Burnout

Burnout reveals itself in all aspects of your life. I've talked about some of the signs that are most conspicuous because they reveal themselves externally, through your key relationships. But the most devastating toll occurs internally, in your own mind and body: predictable emotional and physical symptoms of a condition that is disease-like in its specificity.

Emotional Signs of Burnout

As a guy, I can neither confirm nor deny that I have ever experienced a feeling. Doing so would be a violation of the GUY CODE, and I would be subject to fines and other punishment if I made such an admission. However, since it's just you and me here, I'll tell you in confidence that, while burning out, I frequently felt frustrated, negative, cynical, out of control, listless, angry, and moody. Even worse, I did not talk about these feelings or even admit to myself that I had them. Instead, I simply swallowed them and let them stew. Yes, it's a guy thing. But then again, it's a woman thing too. I know a lot of women who were brought up to put on a happy face no matter what the circumstances. I am married to, and deeply in love with, such a woman. I spent the first five years of our relationship trying to read her mind so I would know what she really thought and felt; it didn't work. It took a long time for me to realize I wasn't clairvoyant and for her to discover she could take off the happy-face mask, be herself, and still be loved.

Our society has a number of ways of encouraging us to hide our true feelings and fall out of touch with our inner selves. These make it easy to become blind to the emotional warning signs of burnout. We tend to have more practice repressing and ignoring feelings than we do recognizing them, naming them, and taking appropriate action.

Here is a list that providers have shared with me over the last few years of the most common feelings associated with stress and burnout. As you read through the list, think about your own feelings and see if you've experienced any of them recently.

- ◄ Apathy/emptiness

- ◄ Anxiety/nervousness

- ◄ Frustration

- ◄ Sadness

- ◄ Depression

- ◄ Anger/irritability

- ◄ Negativity/cynicism

- ◄ Pessimism

- ◄ Volatility/overreaction

- ◄ Strong fears or phobias

- ◄ Powerlessness/passivity

If you are going to avoid or recover from burnout, you need to learn how to recognize the feelings that lead up to and cause it. Then you need to get in touch with the internal and external stressors that lead in that direction. You have to learn to name the hurt, identify the trouble, and feel the pain. Each is an important step in the process of learning to care for yourself.

Physical Signs of Burnout

Some people are so good at ignoring their feelings that their bodies have to kick things up a notch to get their attention. Are you one of them? If you listen, it can tell you when you need to change the way you live. Unresolved mental unrest definitely manifests itself in physical ways. How many of the following symptoms do you carry around with you during the day?

- Back, shoulder, and neck tightness or pain
- Chronic headaches
- Immune system problems resulting in more colds, flu, and infections
- Unhealthy eating habits
- Eating disorders
- Addictive behaviors
- Constipation, diarrhea, or other gastrointestinal problems
- Skin problems (hives, eczema, psoriasis, itching)
- Tics
- Nervous stomach
- Sleep problems
- Poor memory/poor concentration
- Reproductive problems

◄ High blood pressure

◄ Lack of energy/fatigue

◄ Hair loss

◄ Teeth grinding/other periodontal problems

These are some of the most common physical and behavioral signs that you are not making healthy life choices. You are not alone: every time I talk with providers about burnout, these are the signals that become part of the discussion. Unaddressed feelings of stress and burnout can become so severe that your body starts to fall apart.

Looking back on my own burnout experience, I realize that although my blood pressure was perfect, I never had headaches, and I hardly ever caught a cold, my body was nonetheless sending me signals. My back, or some other muscle group, was always aching, my energy levels steadily dropped, and I ate terribly. The good news is that I finally started to listen to all of these signals. The bad news is that it took six years or so for me to hear them, and another two years before I started making changes. Take the time to sit down fully in tune with your physical self and listen to what it is telling you. The longer you ignore the signals, the harder it will be to make the needed changes. Failure to listen to yourself may ultimately result in serious health problems.

When It Is More Than Burnout

In *Overcoming Job Burnout*, Beverly Potter has written, "As the occupational 'blahs' become chronic, many burnouts seek chemical solutions to overwhelming emotional demands and stresses. People often drink more alcohol, eat more or eat less and use drugs such as sleeping pills, tranquilizers, and mood elevators. Chain smoking and drinking large amounts of coffee and sugar are also common. This increased substance abuse further compounds health problems." As a community center director, I once had to fire an employee because he was drinking before work to "take the edge off." Later, when I was a center director, I had to terminate a young woman who was smoking weed in the parking lot during her break. There was a story in the news recently of a provider arrested for drunk driving—in a fifteen-passenger van full of children. Burnout can leave some caregivers feeling so empty that they look for quick ways to fill themselves up and feel good for a while. What were just escape activities can blossom into serious disorders such as chemical dependency; overeating; and compulsive behaviors including shopping, gambling, and sex. Dealing with burnout-related behavior this severe is beyond the scope of this book. I urge providers who feel they may have addiction problems to seek professional help. If you know a provider who has an addiction problem, do what you can to ensure her safety and the safety of the children in her care.

Why We Burn Out—The Ten Chief Contributors to Burnout

As many reasons for provider burnout exist as there are providers. The following list includes the ten most common contributors to burnout, but feel free to add your own.

- ◢ Caring for everyone but yourself

- ◢ Working for limited rewards and appreciation

- ◢ Not seeing the payoff

- ◢ Children leaving your program

- ◢ Isolation

- ◢ Inadequate income

- ◢ Heavy workload

- ◢ Excessive physical demands

◢ Repetitiveness

◢ Powerlessness and helplessness

Do you see your triggers anywhere in this list? If so, read on for more details.

Caring for Everyone but Yourself

What happens if you give a child care provider a canteen full of water and send him off to cross a desert? He dies of thirst because he stops to water every cactus and give drinks to each coyote, rattle-snake, and scorpion he encounters.

Probably the number-one contributor to burnout is your habit of spending more time and energy caring for others than you do caring for yourself—probably *lots* more. To see if this is true of you, grab paper and a pen and complete this two-part exercise:

1. List all the things you have done for others in the last seven days; include anything and everything you've done for someone other than yourself. Take your time; make a thorough list. If you do not have time to do it all in one sitting, come back to your list throughout the day as you think of things to add. There is no reason to rush. But however long it takes you, *don't read past this paragraph until you have taken the time to complete this step*.

2. For the second part of the activity, write down everything you did for yourself in the same seven days. Include only things you did *just for yourself*. Take all the time you need.

If you are anything like the hundreds of providers with whom I have completed this exercise, your first list will be much longer than the second. The problem this identifies permeates caregiving professions, including professional child care: caregivers commit much more time and energy to taking care of others than to taking care of themselves. When I give providers five minutes during trainings to fill an index card with all the things they did for other people, they have no problem filling the entire card. Someone always jokes that she needs an entire package of cards. I've seen some people write so fast that their pens almost burst into flame. It's no big surprise: caregivers take care of people—that's your job. Heck, it's even in the job title. As caregivers, you wipe noses, tie shoes, cover the hours of your coworkers, make meals, mentor peers, drive anyone anywhere, change diapers, skip breaks, listen, empathize, care for physical and emotional wounds, share yourself, and do almost anything else that anyone wants.

Yet when I ask providers to fill the second card with the things they have done for themselves, the training room gets so quiet you could hear a snail hiccup. Participants hem and haw as they squirm in their seats. They jot down one thing, maybe two. They chew their lips and soon give up trying to think of anything else. A few can share what they wrote: exercise, shopping, having a beer and relaxing, talking with a friend. In every session, someone always writes, "I took a shower." Now, I understand that a long hot shower can be very refreshing and energizing. I know it may represent your only time alone all day. But when personal hygiene is the only activity you make time to give yourself, you are *really* not making enough time for yourself. Many providers cannot name a single activity they undertook for themselves in a week's time. This is tragic, and not only because you're shortchanging yourself: by failing to take care of yourself, you are also limiting your ability to care for others effectively. Sooner or later, you will become empty, used up, and worn out.

Look at your own list. What does it say about how you apportion your time? What does it say about your priorities? Is it surprising that you are stressed, strained, and stretched too thin? Can you see why you might be a candidate for burnout?

It isn't surprising that providers end up physically and emotionally drained from caring for others; most of you who gravitate toward care-giving professions are naturally empathic. You can easily get in touch with the feelings of the people around you, and you're sympathetic and sensitive to their needs. The upside of such inborn empathy is that you can easily get in tune with the individual children in your care; you know how to effectively lead the dance that goes on be-tween yourself and a child. And in turn, this ability assures that each child gets the unique care her personality and circumstances requires. The downside is merely the flipside of that strength: you know how to dance emotionally with many different people—children, parents of those children (and often stepparents, grandparents, and other family members), coworkers and peers, and your own family—and their many different needs, expectations, and abilities to respond. Because by the nature of your job you are required to tune in to the emotional state of these dance partners, too often you take on some of their emotional baggage. It is a lot like one of those old episodes of *Star Trek* where the very rational, nonemotional Vulcan, Mr. Spock, does a mind-meld in which he lays his hand on some alien creature's head and reads its thoughts and feelings. Spock ends up physically and emotionally ex-hausted, depleted from learning all there is to know about the crea-ture and feeling all the feelings that the creature feels.

Something similar happens to child care providers all the time: you end up carrying around the emotional detritus of dozens of people. When this load is added to your failure to care for yourself, you end up emotionally drained, physically exhausted, and danced out.

Working for Limited Rewards and Appreciation

For my thirty-seventh birthday, two kids in our care, Jack and Sam (with some help from their mom), gave me a bag of Reese's Peanut Butter Cups, a bag of Twizzlers, and the book *Apples for a Teacher*. As I paged through the book, munching peanut butter cups, I came across a poem that starts:

It's not so much what we say
As the manner in which we say it.
It's not so much the language we use
As the tone in which we convey it.
      (author unknown, "The Tone of Voice")

The candy was great, but I will forever cherish those words and the book, especially the inscription, which thanked me for being a good provider and mentor for the boys. Working as a professional provider of early care and education can be emotionally fulfilling and rewarding. Consider the many wonderful benefits: the hugs, the smiles, the knowledge that you are having a positive impact on children's futures. Gifts like the ones I received from Jack and Sam brighten my day, lift my spirit, and fill my soul. It feels good to be appreciated.

Sadly, not all providers feel appreciated and valued by the families they work with, their workplaces, and their communities.

As a child care provider, you work long hours in isolation, and you rarely receive feedback on the quality of your work. When you do, as often as not what you get is complaints or criticism. Not knowing how you are doing at your job often contributes to burnout; it's hard to stay fresh and energized when you do not know how well you are performing. Most programs fail to build adequate systems for collecting feedback on providers' performance, and most providers do not seek out feedback. This makes it very difficult to know what you are doing right and wrong. What changes are needed so that you can operate more effectively?

It's hard to do a job well when feedback is limited. If you're a family child care provider, unless you belong to an association or peer-support group, usually you don't receive any peer feedback at all. Sometimes providers are too meek to ask, "How am I doing?" Other times, the work environment is to blame: either by design or omission, the work setting is not a place in which information flows freely. Either way, when you don't receive clear and regular feedback, burnout cannot be far away.

As if being underappreciated isn't enough, most of you are grossly underpaid. You probably knew going in that caregiving, while enriching in so many ways, was not going to make you rich. Your fellow providers have repeatedly cited wages and benefits as the reasons they have chosen to leave the profession. For many of you, benefits such as health insurance, paid vacations, and sick time are nonexistent. I know providers who have gone nearly a decade without a pay increase, who go to work sick because they can't afford to take an unpaid day off, and who have missed family weddings and funerals because they are unable to get away from their jobs.

And yet, many providers say that the benefit they desire most is a regular daily break. For some of you, it's difficult even to find a few minutes to go to the bathroom. If you work in a center, you probably have to wait to take a bathroom break until another caregiver shows up to watch the children. If you work out of your own home, you have to find the strategically right moment to rush to the bathroom, then cope with the knocks, calls, and fingers waving under the door while you are relieving yourself.

Think about it: What other professions can you name in which the work actually follows you into the bathroom? There are very few careers in which an uninterrupted trip to the bathroom is considered a job benefit. Yet for many caregivers, the breaks and lunch *hours* their friends in other professions talk about are purely mythic. Think about that: an entire *hour,* or even a *half* hour, of peace in which to eat, relax, and run an errand or two. For too many child care providers, this is only a daydream. It's not difficult to imagine becoming burned out when you can't remember your last break or leisurely visit to the bathroom. (One home provider I know began to understand how much her husband understood and respected what she did during the day when he started coming home on his lunch hour to spend time with the kids so she could use the bathroom, eat her lunch, and have a few moments of solitude in the middle of the day. This kind of understanding and appreciation is rare.) Society—even family members—tends to view providers as babysitters, not as early care and education professionals. While some people realize how difficult and demanding early care and education is, many others dismiss it as "a job where you stay at home and watch TV all day." That is one prevalent myth—that providers sit around, watch *Oprah*, and eat bonbons while the children quietly play in a corner. Too many people do not view the work of child care providers as real professional work. This affects you: it's difficult to feel proud of your career choice when society does not hold it in high esteem.

Not Seeing the Payoff

Even with the debilitating effects of poor pay, paltry benefits, lack of appreciation, and little feedback, providers might feel prouder of their work if they had a clearer connection to what they accomplish. People who work in a factory making widgets see a stack of shiny new widgets at the end of each day. People who construct buildings see daily progress, and a house, hotel, or hospital rises as the end result of their labor. In contrast, providers rarely see their finished product: they seldom see the adults those children become. I do know some providers who have cared for multiple generations of the same family, nurturing and educating the children of children they cared for twenty years ago. They have strong bonds and regular contact over long spans of time. But this happens infrequently; providers and families tend to drift apart, losing contact as their lives unfold.

Most children do not remember the providers who cared for them during their precious formative years. You know you make a difference in the life of every child you work with—but knowing that *they* know you touched their lives would also be very rewarding. Will Jack keep his love of bugs and have a show on *Animal Planet*? Will Maddie still wear colorful ribbons in her flame-red hair and detest sand between her toes when she turns thirty? Ginger moved away before she turned two—does she still have that devilish grin and that gleam in her eyes? Will Hunter drive a pickup truck and be a cop? Will these children become happy, successful, and fulfilled adults? Will they remember the hours and hours they spent in my home and heart? Will they remember me?

In the last photograph I took of Ginger, she sat smiling under a blanket that Tasha had crocheted for her. It was her last day in our program before moving back to Florida. She came into our home when she was about six weeks old. It takes a lot of work to tune in to some kids, a huge investment of time and energy. Ginger wasn't one of those kids. We clicked as soon as we met. We shared smiles, hugs, first step, and first words. She stole my heart.

Then her family moved to Florida.

Not knowing what becomes of the children you care for can be emotionally unsettling. You give them so much of yourself that it would be nice to know what kinds of people they turn into as they grow and mature. Time and distance separate you from the payoff for your hard work. You care for, love, and shape the child, but the adult is usually unknown to you.

Children Leaving Your Program

It's 5:50 AM on February 27. Fair-skinned, redheaded, inquisitive, funny, empathetic, smart, almost-four-year-old Maddie arrived about twenty minutes ago. We haven't seen her for two weeks because her family is in the process of moving to Fargo, North Dakota. Mom has started her new job there. Dad and Maddie are staying in Sioux City until they sell the old house and buy a new one. With her mother gone, Maddie will be getting to our house about this time for the next few weeks so Dad can make it to work on time. Maddie and I are sitting in the playroom talking by the light of the aquarium: "We're moving to Fargo . . . but not yet," she confides.

"Yes, as soon as you sell your old house and buy a new house, you will move to Fargo."

"Will you miss me?"

"I will miss you very much. I have known you since you were a tiny baby. I will be very sad when you move."

"I will miss you and Tasha very much too."

We sit and cuddle, enjoying our time together, knowing it won't last much longer.

This is a conversation Maddie and I have shared often over the last five or six weeks, preparing ourselves for this big transition. Maddie has spent between 10 and 15 percent of her first four years in our care. She became part of our family, her warm smile brightening our lives. A few weeks after this conversation, she would be gone, and there would be another hole in my heart.

Children leaving programs can be a huge stressor. Providers invest enormous amounts of emotional capital building strong connections with children and then, inevitably, the kids move on. They start school, they move out of town, they change programs, and sometimes they just disappear without a good-bye because they are part of their parents' chaotic lives. Whatever the reason, kids leave, and we are left to fill the void. I'm man enough to admit that Maddie's departure caused an allergy attack that made my eyes water for a while . . . Okay, I cried. I still get misty-eyed when I think about her departure. It was the same with Ginger and so many others. Such departures leave holes in my heart that are slow to heal. Building relationships is exhausting, and losing them is painful.

Yet building strong, meaningful relationships with the children who enter your program is part of the job. And so is learning how to let go and helping the children and their families make the transition. The authentic relationships you build are the foundation for early learning, and building that foundation helps set the children on their life's journey. You cannot do your job right without getting close to the children, and you can't fake it. You can't keep them from growing up and moving on. The feelings of loss that come with children leaving your program are inevitable, as is the pain that burnout causes when you don't learn to acknowledge and express those feelings, along with all the other emotions your daily struggles call up.

Isolation

Whether you work in a center or a family-based program, isolation is a problem for you as a provider. You spend your entire day with children and have very limited, usually brief, contact with other adults. Coping with limited adult contact is difficult for many providers. In most settings, workers can share ideas, concerns, frustrations, dreams, and gossip with coworkers and colleagues. They build friendships and bonds. Working with other adults has its difficulties, of course, but it can be therapeutic and rewarding on many levels. Such relationships are difficult to build in many child care programs, where contact with other adults is minimal.

Social isolation is an important cause of burnout, especially for rural, home-based providers. For most of the week, their lives are confined by the walls of their home, cutting them off from the outside world. Many feel "stuck in a box" without contact with the "real world." Imagine spending every workday of a long midwestern winter ten miles from town caring for eight children under age five. Just the idea of such isolation is enough to stress some people. Some non-providers may think it sounds idyllic—sitting with the kids, all cozy and warm, while the winter wind rattles the window. The fact is, such work is hard, and the stress caused by isolation is often overpowering—a prime breeding ground for anxiety and burnout.

This came to me by e-mail from a provider named Connie: "I suspect a lot of burnout comes from being so isolated in our jobs. We only get to interact with children for the majority of our days. No matter how much fun you have with the kids, you always crave adult conversation with someone who doesn't ask *Why?* every other word."

Daily isolation from other adults is not the only isolation providers must deal with. In many ways, you are isolated simply by working in this field. Not a lot of people understand what it is that you do. This lack of understanding marginalizes providers as professionals, isolating you from other educators, helping professionals, and social service providers. Caregivers are rarely invited to the table when social, economic, education, and other issues are discussed by those with power. This lack of contact, this segregation, leads to feelings of loneliness and devalues the importance of what you do.

Inadequate Income

The Wilder Research Center report I mentioned in chapter 2 found that 67 percent of center and preschool staff rated dissatisfaction with wages as their top reason for leaving the profession. The numbers were not much better for other kinds of early childhood programs: 63 percent of Head Start workers, 56 percent of school-age caregivers, and 32 percent of family providers rated meager income as their primary reason for leaving the field.

I've never met a provider who entered the field expecting to get rich. In most programs, pay increases are small and infrequent, and this fact is seldom hidden from new caregivers. People enter the field fully aware that the wages will be low. Yet they still enter the field. Some do it out of necessity; they need a job now, and any job will do. Many more enter the field because the calling to work with children is so strong that they trick themselves into believing that somehow wages and other extrinsic rewards will improve, or they knowingly choose to sacrifice and live on their small incomes. Other workers take entry-level positions in preschools or centers at low wages with the intention of working their way up the ranks through a combination of experience and additional schooling.

Each of these categories of provider can become burned out. Many find that the workload is physically and psychologically taxing, not worth the poor wages. Some find that they love the job but are unable to live on the pay. They don't feel that paying their dues by getting the schooling necessary to improve their status is worth it. Sometimes they recognize that acquiring such status would come at the price of an administrative position that would take them away from children, when working with kids was the very thing that attracted them to the work. Over time, very few providers manage to find a way to make a decent living on providers' wages.

Heavy Workload

The pay is poor, but at least the workload is heavy. People who think child care is an easy job need to spend a few weeks living the life of a provider. Giving children a safe, healthy, nurturing, engaging, loving, and friendly environment is not easy. On top of that there are paperwork, cleaning, planning, and a thousand more details that demand your attention. Child care is a mentally *and* physically challenging job by anyone's standards. Whether you work part-time in a center-based program or sixty hours or more a week as a family child care provider, the job is downright exhausting. On top of this, many full-time providers must work second jobs to make ends meet.

The long hours and the intensity of the work can be very fulfilling if you believe that you are making a difference in the lives of the children—but as I've already observed, this isn't always the case. And unless you learn ways to take care of yourself, you may come to spend too many of your days feeling run-down and worn-out, living for the weekends, dreaming of the end of the day, and wishing for a job that doesn't demand so much.

For many providers, one of the toughest challenges comes on the weekend or the rare day off. Such times are too often filled with caring for family members and meeting family obligations. Many providers burn out because they carry the weight of the world on their shoulders, twenty-four hours a day, seven days a week. They never find time to lay their burden down and rest, stretch, and breathe.

Excessive Physical Demands

Caring for young children is physically demanding. During a recent school break, for example, we had extra school-age kids in the house. They wanted to chill out, talk, and build with Legos. We built and built and built: houses, cars, spaceships. Three hours later, my back was killing me. It has happened before and it will happen again—I have Lego back. Carrying babies, toting toddlers, chasing preschoolers, and herding school-age children is a lot of work. So is serving meals, crawling around on your hands and knees, and all the other heaving and ho-ing we do. Many people who enter the field are unprepared for the physical demands of the profession. They soon find that they are unequipped for the hard work and leave the field. Others survive for a long time before sore backs, stiff necks, and creaky knees catch up with them. The heavy lifting that child care demands can lead to exhaustion if providers do not make adjustments to deal with physical strain.

Repetitiveness

Renae, a provider from South Dakota, shared this in an e-mail: "We perform the same tasks day after day, some of them very menial, such as diaper changes, lunch preparation, and shoe-tying. After repeatedly following the same routine day after day after day, our brains go on automatic pilot. We can do our jobs without even thinking." Like many jobs, child care involves a lot of repetition. This can become yet another source of stress for providers for whom the challenges of child care are already outweighing the rewards. While refreshed and energized providers are eager to try new activities and handle situations differently, providers who are overtaxed by repetition may become even more repetitive once they narrow their range of responses, in turn making their jobs even more stressful. Looking at recurring responsibilities and duties with fresh eyes is hard enough to do in the best of times; it's almost impossible when you're run down to the point of burnout.

Powerlessness and Helplessness

Each of the factors in burnout that I've mentioned so far contributes to the feelings of powerlessness and helplessness that figure prominently in the profession. The poor pay, long hours, hard work, and limited appreciation weigh down on those of us who are willing to stay in the field, leaving many feeling powerless and helpless. Such providers are physically and emotionally unable to make needed changes; they stay in the profession because they are emotionally stuck—they truly feel they have no other choices. Inevitably their job performance suffers and the quality of care they provide substantially diminishes, but still they hang on until they crash—or worse, until they're forced out by poor performance or complaints from parents.

If you're one of those providers who feels powerless and stuck, you can make steady, subtle changes to break this cycle if you really want to stay in this profession and are willing to make the effort. Unhappily, too many providers have become so jaded, cynical, and exhausted that they will never fully regain their passion for early care and education. For their sakes and those of the children in their care, it's best for them to move on and try something else.

The Many Faces of Denial

Providers tend to put on different masks when facing the situations contributing to their stress. They may deny that they may be burning out—strong faces, stoic faces, sarcastic faces, glib faces, happy faces, in-control faces, and countless others. They try to look as if they are still fully in the game, still enthusiastic, even though their enthusiasm may have flagged long ago. Providers may spend years behind these masks, trying to hide their impending burnout from the world—and themselves.

To deal effectively with burnout, you must remove all the masks and address head-on the feelings and issues that you have denied or avoided. You must find ways to become comfortable in your own skin again, to renew your love of the profession, and to refresh your attitude.

Do We Implode or Explode?

What happens when burnout finally reaches its crisis point varies from person to person, but I believe there are two basic styles of burn-out: you implode or you explode.

Imploders tend to internalize all of their stresses and pressures, living with them, nurturing them, almost befriending them. Imploders tend to keep all their frustrations, worries, stress, anxiety, and tension inside for as long as they can. These are the people who are more likely to feel powerless and helpless, believing they can't change their situation and that no one is capable of helping. On some level, they know they are burning out. They can feel it building for a long time; they can see their patience dwindling, their energy draining, their creativity waning, and their stress increasing. They may quietly and indirectly ask for help, but not in a way that allows people outside their situation to realize how much they are suffering. Instead, they

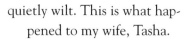

quietly wilt. This is what happened to my wife, Tasha.

Exploders, on the other hand, seem actually to *thrive* on their stresses and pressures, spreading them around and increasing them. They don't even seem to realize that stress and pressure are negative and are hurting them—for a while anyway. Exploders feed on stress and pressure and freely share it with others. They tend not to see their own burnout until it's almost too late to do anything constructive about it. They think they are handling their stress just fine—and then one day—*boom!* they burst, burning out in a dazzling display of flames. I exploded.

Whether you are burning out with a bang or a whimper, the following chapters offer you strategies for dealing with stressful environments so that you can make some steady, subtle, and crucial changes in your life that can steer you away from burnout, and move you toward more manageable and rewarding work. Too many experienced and skilled providers leave the early care and education profession because they don't know how to recognize and deal with the inherent stresses of this demanding work. You don't need to become one of them.

Setting the Stage for Mindful Change

Take the time to reflect on and complete the following exercise. Doing so will help you recognize and deal with the causes of your burnout. You need to know *what* is burning you out before you can change it. Grab some paper and a pen and write down your answers to these questions:

1. What three things do you enjoy most about your work, and why?

2. What three things about your work environment cause you the most stress, and why?

3. What three things would you change about your work environment, and why? (Note that these aren't necessarily the three things that cause you the most stress!)

4. What three recurring nonenvironmental situations or events cause you the most stress, and why?

5. What three subtle changes *in yourself* could you make to reduce your stress, and why?

6. Which three people in your life cause you the most stress, and why?

Now take a *really* deep breath and answer this REALLY BIG question (more about this and the other questions later).

7. What do you believe your Ultimate Purpose is in life, and why?

Be honest and thorough. Then spend some time with your answers. Reflect on what you wrote; get to know especially the *why* of what you wrote. Your answers to these questions reveal a lot about what is going on in your life and head. They will help prepare you for the work to come.

REFERENCES

Maslach, Christina. 2003. *Burnout: The Cost of Caring*. Cambridge, Mass.: Malor Books/ISHK.

Potter, Beverly. 2005. *Overcoming Job Burnout: How to Renew Enthusiasm for Work*. Oakland, Calif.: Ronin Publishing.

Reece, Colleen, and Anita Corinne Donihue, eds. 2002. *Apples for a Teacher: A Bushel of Stories, Poems, and Prayers*. Uhrichsville, Ohio: Barbour Publishing.

Time Out

Stress-Reducing Inventions for Providers

Wouldn't life as a provider be peachy if someone took the time to invent a few gadgets to make the job easier? Well, for your benefit, and the benefit of all humankind, I have thought up the following inventions to help you get through your workdays more efficiently and less stressfully. As far as I know, none of these items are currently on the market. Don't tell anyone, but I have a top-notch team of early education innovators and engineers working on prototypes in a secret lab located inside a dormant volcano somewhere in the South Pacific. We hope to begin beta testing in a few years and to unveil the first commercial units in the spring of 2015 during the National Association for the Education of Young Children conference. The products will be costly, but they should be fully deductible as business expenses.

Pneumatic Child Delivery System

Drop-off and pickup time can be the most stressful times of day for providers. Parents are rushed, kids act up, and you feel as if you can't pay enough attention to everyone during the hurried comings and goings. The Pneumatic Child Delivery Tube is the answer. Imagine a gigantic version of the air-powered tubes used at drive-through banks: one end in your driveway, the other in your playroom. Children simply climb into the clear plastic canisters and zip into your house or out to their parent's car. *Whoooooosh!* They enjoy the ride, and you enjoy stress-free transition time.

Secretion-Eating Nanobots

Do you ever feel as if you're drowning in snot, drool, dirty diapers, and other childish secretions? Some tiny little noses drip snot like Niagara Falls rains water; some kids drool so much they leave slick and slimy trails . . . as if they were gigantic, fast-moving mutant snails. The elephantine piles of foul-smelling poo created by some angelic-looking children would make Beelzebub himself blush. This is why the lab is developing Secretion-Eating Nanobots. The microscopic nanobots are designed to scurry around child care programs, devouring all the foul fluids and solids that leak out of children throughout the day. Hundreds of miniature, nearly invisible robots swarm to each soiled diaper and runny nose almost before the mess is made. They keep everyone cleaner, healthier, and happier.

(Within an hour of writing the paragraph above, a wonderful little five-month-old we care for peed all over me and urped up part of a bottle while I was changing his diaper. I've told the lab that this project is high priority.)

Eyes-in-the-Back-of-the-Head Implant

Many children think adults have eyes in the back of their heads. Won't it be nice when you really do? A same-day surgical procedure, these ocular implants give you a 360-degree view of any room. You can immediately spot the trouble that usually starts as soon as you turn your head. The implants can be upgraded to include optical zoom capability and digital video recording so you can make a record of everything that happens.

Expandable Lap

Most people are looking for ways to keep their laps from expanding, but nothing would be better for reading with children than a lap roomy enough to accommodate six or eight small people. At our house, when an adult sits on the floor, a line of kids holding books instantly forms. Pushing matches often occur to get the coveted front-row-center seat on the lap. The Expandable Lap clips onto the user's hips and thighs, creating a comfortable seating area for multiple children. It comes with viewing screens and cuddle cushions, so each child can feel as if she is the only one on your lap.

Super-Duper Utility Belt

Batman has one, Wonder Woman has one—why not you? Need rubber gloves and a Band-Aid? Reach into your utility belt. Need a facial tissue? Grab one from your utility belt. Need glue, scissors, washable markers, and a few sheets of paper? Check the belt. The keys to the super-duper utility belt are compartmentalization and micro-technology. This belt holds tons of stuff made as small as possible, and because everything is so well organized, you won't accidentally pull out a baby T-Rex when what you're really reaching for is water toys.

Child care providers are unsung real-life superheroes and should at least get to look the part. Kids will view you with awe and respect when they see you in your new titanium-plated utility belt and diamond-studded cape!

Holographic Activity Room

Your holographic activity room replicates any desired setting, using supercomputers and virtual-reality technology. You can take the kids to the beach when it is ten below zero, you can all visit the zoo without worrying about lost children or sunburn—or even leaving the house. You can let them fool around in the mud without a huge mess to clean up after play. Just turn on the computer, program the setting, and send the kids off to enjoy themselves.

Robot Maid

As a child, I believed that by the time I was an adult, all families would have their own household robots to do all the tasks we humans are too busy to complete. After all, George Jetson had Rosie, the Robinson family had Robot (not much of a name), and Luke Skywalker had R2-D2. What child care providers need is helpful robots to pick up toys, take out trash, mop floors, do paperwork, make simple repairs, and maybe wash windows now and then. They will give us more time with the kids and cut a lot of drudgery from the caregiving day.

Jetpack

I have wanted a jetpack since seeing James Bond use one in the opening sequence of the movie *Thunderball*. I think it would be a great gadget for child care providers. You may not need it every day, but it would be perfect for quick trips to the store for groceries in the morning or for errands during a break. It would also come in handy for retrieving Frisbees from rooftops, returning windblown baby birds to their nests, and assisting kittens and small children out of trees. I also guarantee that as jetpack use increases in child care, so will the number of men working in the field.

The above inventions would certainly be useful, and they're fun to think about. While they might help reduce your stress level and workload in some ways, they would probably lead to fresh problems and anxiety in others. What if the pneumatic tube malfunctioned, or the nanobots went berserk? The expandable lap might be more efficient, but story time wouldn't be as cozy. Virtual-reality mud might not require cleanup, but it would also probably lack the ooey-gooeyness of the real thing.

In the end, we have to look inward for the solutions to our stresses. If we want to change our lives, we have to change our minds and realign our thinking. Bliss does not come from having more things; it comes from having a deeper relationship with ourselves, a truer vision of who we really are.

4

Changing Your Mind (Literally) and Taking Action

You do not like them.
So you say.
Try them! Try them!
And you may.
Try them and you may, I say.

—Sam-I-Am, in Dr. Seuss's *Green Eggs and Ham*

SAM'S UNNAMED BUDDY in the Dr. Seuss classic *Green Eggs and Ham* is a lot like most of us: set in his ways and reluctant to try anything new. We are generally so content with the status quo that we even take some sort of odd comfort in the uncomfortable, painful, stressful, agonizing parts of our lives. I guarantee that you know someone (or perhaps you are that someone?) who makes friends with his troubles, nurturing them, feeding them, stroking them behind the ears, sharing pictures with friends of how those troubles have grown.

"Great to see you, Cassie! It's been too long. I'm so glad we've found time to catch up. How are you?"

"Oh, I know it's been too long. . . . I've missed seeing you too. I've been working eight-hour days at the center, sometimes nine or ten. The kids have been driving me crazy. . . . I think it's the weather. The director has hired some new staff members . . . a couple of young kids from the college. They're nice but can't always work

when she wants, and someone has to cover the toddler room. The licensing people were by last week, investigating a complaint. Enrollment is down. I think I'm getting the flu. . . . Something has been going around. My cat is sick. When I finally do get home at night, it seems like I have a day's work to do just to keep the house in order and the family on track. They try to help but don't do things the way they are supposed to. I've been feeling so stressed. I'm not sleeping. I've had a headache since last June. The dog puked on my new . . ."

On and on the litany goes; the things that stress us out become part of the family. We are all creatures of comfortable habit. Change is often anything but easy. Who wants to try something new when you are perfectly content (or content being *unhappy*) with the way things are? People have their favorite chairs, T-shirts, and pizza toppings, so why not favorite problems and excuses for not trying new things? You probably aren't looking for anything new—not in a box with a fox, in a house with a mouse, or anywhere else, for that matter.

Cocoa and the Human Brain

This brings us to hot chocolate, nectar of the gods. Sometimes it gets cold in our little corner of northwestern Iowa, and nothing tastes better than a cup of hot chocolate. Tasha and I have tried every blend of hot chocolate from every hot chocolate machine in every convenience store and restaurant in town. Once we had found the best-tasting stuff, we made a habit of going to that particular gas station every time the cocoa bug struck. One of the families in our program bought us a hot chocolate maker for Christmas one year, but we haven't been able to blend a brew of our own that matches the stuff from that gas station. So for years during the winter, I often found myself trudging out into the snow and wind, cleaning off the van, and driving to get two cups of the right cocoa. It was okay, though: we had found cocoa we liked, and life was good.

That is, until one morning when I walked in for my usual pair of twenty-ounce cups and noticed that Rosie, the store manager—someone I have known since middle school—dropped her eyes as soon as I walked up to the counter. I knew something was up. I looked past the donut display and gum rack to the beverage corner, and there saw something to make my heart sink. The reliable old hot chocolate machine, an essential part of our winter routine for so many years, was *gone*. A shiny new espresso-mocha-latte-spewing contraption now sat in its place. I had to sweep my jaw up off the floor.

How would I explain this to Tasha? Then I came to my senses. Just because the machine was different didn't necessarily mean the beverage would be. In fact, it was possible that the new cocoa would taste even better than the brew we loved.

It wasn't, of course—it was too watery, had an icky after-taste, and . . . well, it just wasn't *our* cocoa, the stuff we enjoyed on snowy winter mornings or at the beginning of long road trips. It was basically the same brew, but it tasted annoyingly different. There we were, stranded in the deep of an Iowa winter without the perfect hot chocolate. Someday we may find a new favorite, but we will never forget the dark frothy cocoa we loved so much.

All of this may sound silly, but the change of cocoa machines forced us to change some of our habits, and these had included one of our marriage rituals:

"Would you like some cocoa?" I would ask as we got ready for the day.

"If you're getting yourself some," she would respond.

"I'm not going to go just for myself, but if you want some, I'll have some too."

And on it went, until I walked out the door after the drinks. It was something so simple, but so nice, so soothing.

Now, if changing something as trivial as your cocoa can be

traumatic, making bigger changes across your entire life can seem completely overwhelming.

Our Brains and Minds Can Change

We have to face it: you and I aren't children anymore. Our minds are harder to change both physically and intellectually. We're set in our ways, although a growing body of scientific evidence says that people can continue to change, no matter how old we become or how ingrained our habits.

Each of us has millions of pathways called *synapses* that connect the nerve cells in our brains. Brain pathways that get used regularly remain in good repair, throbbing with chemo-electric traffic. Unused pathways, on the other hand, get pruned away. These pathways manifest themselves physically in our habits. When I thought "GO GET COCOA," my brain snapped to attention, remembering the directions to the convenience store, where my keys were, the temperature outside, and my need for a jacket. My mouth started to water because it was getting signals that a treat was coming. My entire body went into action.

Our habits are programmed into us at a cellular level. Even so, we old dogs can be taught new tricks. We just have to trade in our dingy old habits for thoughtful new ones; we have to reprogram our brains. Humans are lucky enough to be blessed with something called neuroplasticity, the brain's innate ability to transform itself physically to deal with things like injury, new information, and stimulation. The brain, in other words, is flexible and adaptable. The landscape of our brains changes over time. Just like an old footpath, brain connections that don't get used much can eventually be erased, leaving no signs that they ever existed. The pathways that get used a lot remain vivid and instantly accessible. Happily, new pathways are always being made.

The children we care for are all about neuroplasticity. During those first five years of life, their brains grow and adapt at incredible rates. They are constantly changing as they play, explore, and discover the world.

Part of our job as early care and education professionals is to make sure that these children receive the developmentally appropriate stimulation their growing brains need. We feed them nutritious meals, provide them with learning materials, and model good behavior. Even more important, we help them develop good physical and mental habits. To do so, we need to remain as flexible and curious as we can possibly be too.

To Boldly Go Where No One Has Gone Before

I have written about how it's sometimes easier to live with stress, malaise, and trouble than to make changes and step boldly into the unknown. It's easy to get stuck in ruts, allowing health problems, aches and pains, marital troubles, work problems, and other stressors to become part—and sometimes practically *all*—of who you are. You can become so comfortable with the status quo (good or bad) that you even become cozy with your burnout-related emotional discomforts. But these start to grow, unnoticed and unchecked, until, with any luck, one day something jars you into becoming aware that you are spinning your wheels and that you just might be better off if you did some things differently. If you hurt badly enough, the idea of change may be less frightening than staying where you are. And that's when you come up against one of the most important lessons you'll ever learn: *Awareness of the problem and acknowledgment that you need to change are the first necessary steps toward change.*

Someone else may be able to open your eyes to your burnout, but transforming your life and changing your habits are both on your shoulders. Change won't happen until you *first become aware of the need for it and then follow that up with a decision to change.* No matter how ingrained your burnout becomes, a voice deep inside is always whispering that things could be different. If you've been contentedly living with your burnout for a long time, you've probably learned to ignore this voice. You muffle it when it says, *The way you're living isn't working.* You suppress its cries for attention. Then, perhaps late one restless night or one afternoon, when four of the eight kids in your care are crying and the other four need their diapers changed, you realize that *something has to change*. You may look in the mirror that evening or the next morning and discover that you don't recognize the person you see. That's when you decide to try something different.

In her book *Transformation Thinking*, Joyce Wycoff wrote, "It is a biological imperative that we grow or die. If we aren't growing, we're dying." We have to grow beyond our burnout. Wycoff noted three types of growth: expanding, extending, and evolving. In the case of burnout, you need to contemplate growing in the following ways:

◄ Expanding your skills, knowledge, and self-awareness

◄ Extending your connections to your inner self as well as to individuals and groups that you find supportive

◄ Evolving into the person you want to be; evolving toward your Ultimate Purpose

This growing awareness of the need to change and this new openness to the possibility for change take place below the surface, transformations that are often invisible to everyone but you. You think about changes you want to make, contemplate what will make you happier, plan how to make time for yourself, and dream of a life free from burnout. The seeds of change must germinate for a while in your fertile mental soil before they can sprout up into the real world of sunlight and air.

A lot of people get to the point of new awareness and new desire to change and then stop. They know they are burned out, and they can identify what led them to that point. They've unmuffled their inner voice and can clearly hear it telling them that life could be better. They have realized that changes need to be made and that they are the ones responsible for making them. They have started changing their minds and are ready to begin changing their worlds. And then, right before their first new buds of growth appear, they stop growing. Their new shoot dies and shrinks back into the mental soil of self.

Many factors can trigger this regression, but in my observations, the two most common factors are *fear* and *guilt*.

Fear and Guilt

Moving from awareness to action can be frightening. People imagine doing all kinds of wonderful things in the privacy of their own minds. They may enjoy contemplating a career change, a return to school, or a new exercise program. These fantasies remain safe as long as they are purely theoretical. In contrast, actually taking the steps to turn those thoughts into reality can be terrifying.

If you find you're afraid to put your thoughts of change into real-world action, you are not alone. It's our old friend: Fear of the Unknown, fear of stepping outside your comfort zone. You don't have to let the fear win. You can take your time, breathe through the fear, and take the first step toward your new life.

Sometimes you have to will yourself past your fears so you can begin the hard work of making healthy changes in your life. This may sound daunting, but moving beyond fear is part of every new learning experience. You move beyond the fear of falling when you take your first steps. You move beyond the fear of not being understood when you first begin to speak. You move beyond the fear of rejection when you make new friends. Your past is full of fears overcome—times when you have moved in new directions and gained new skills.

The other overpowering factor that prevents so many providers from pursuing a burnout-free life is guilt. It is a simple fact that changing your life affects the lives of others. If you take more time to meet your own needs, you have less time to give to the other people in your life. If you say *no* instead of *yes* to requests for your time and energy, the petitioner may feel rejected. You may believe that the changes you make to better your life could have an adverse effect on others. While this is rarely true, it nonetheless makes a lot of caregivers feel guilty. They feel as if they are shirking responsibilities, sidestepping commitments, and leaving people hanging. I felt terribly guilty for a long time after leaving my job as center director; I thought I was disappointing the staff, parents, and kids.

But remember this: people, especially children, benefit from interacting with others who are emotionally and physically healthy and who know how to take care of themselves. If you struggle with guilt, simply accept those feelings as the legacy of your former caregiving self, and let your thoughts of change sprout into real-world action.

Prepare Yourself for Action

Many child care workers feel as if there just isn't enough time in their lives to take the actions required to change from stressed-out to blissed-out. (Well, maybe simply feeling better about ourselves and our work is more realistic. . . .) You may have good intentions, but all too often, you let the busyness of living life get in the way. Books go unread, treadmills become coat racks, bicycles and canoes hang in the garage gathering dust, college applications are completed but never mailed, vacations are planned but never taken, and dreams are dreamed but not lived.

You make excuses, blaming everything from limited time to tired knees, but the reality is that if you could get your mind past the fear of doing, the fear of change, you would find a way to make room in your life for what you want to accomplish. You're the only person who really knows what it will take to change your way of thinking and doing. Whatever tools or techniques you choose to try, please incorporate the following six tips, because your intention and attitude are critical in incorporating changes effectively.

1. *Positive outlook.* The way you think about the world becomes a mirror of the world you live in. If you see the world as dark, dangerous, and dreadful, that is the world in which you will live. If you see a world full of possibilities and potential, that is where you will reside. Thinking positively about situations and people can help you bring about bene-

ficial outcomes; your personal outlook is an important tool in fighting burnout and in changing your thinking.

2. *Self-awareness*. Know who you are. Become aware of your feelings, your breath, your emotions, your thoughts, and your relationships. Know your place in the world so that you can plan for what you would prefer to be. Being self-aware gives you power and control in your life. Start by taking a personal inventory of your traits, good and bad. To know yourself, you have to be comfortable stomping around inside your own head. Examine your life and your past choices. When it comes to facing fears and making changes, you will find, on closer inspection, that you already have the tools, skills, and personal strength to make the changes you need to make. You just need to take a closer look.

3. *Healthy selfishness*. Even though looking after yourself may not come naturally, you need to become comfortable taking care of your own needs. Develop a healthy sense of selfishness so that you can recognize your own needs as valid and do what is necessary to meet them. You've probably spent a lot of time being selfless; now it is time to be a bit selfish.

4. *Relinquish control*. When we are able to relinquish some control and let go of rigid ideas, we become more flexible and better able to change our minds. Life flows better when we can let go. This letting go also allows us to see more options and opportunities in life.

5. *Playful attitude*. Try assuming the attitude of a toddler exploring the world. Changing your mind requires playfulness and good humor, an attitude full of curiosity, whim, and excitement. Allow yourself to become young again and explore your ideas, dreams, thoughts, and fears through a child's eyes.

6. *Thoughtful choices*. Life often becomes so rushed that you either make quick choices that are not well thought out or

put off making choices all together. As you prepare to start making changes in your thinking, slow down enough to make thoughtful, mindful choices. Try to make every choice in your life the best one you can, given what you know at the time. For most people, this takes lots of effort and practice. Reconcile yourself to the fact that you will never entirely master it; give yourself the gift of accepting poor choices from time to time. You must learn to accept that not all of your choices will end with the results you wanted. Better that than never even taking the risk and making the effort. For example, today I've made good choices, like meditation and yoga, and bad choices like too much ice cream and too few vegetables. I try to choose well for me. Sometimes I succeed, sometimes I fail.

Taking Action

As you read and practice the action steps discussed in this chapter, please keep these four guiding principles in mind:

1. *Changes need to be slow, mindful, and well thought out.* If not, they will only add to feelings of burnout. It takes conscious thought, dedication, commitment, and constant effort to transform yourself. You cannot change too quickly; reinventing yourself is a gradual process. It takes time to reprogram your brain.

2. *Seek your truth, find your path.* Everyone is different. Find your own answers and implement them your own way. The suggestions for action that follow are simply that: suggestions. You will be most successful when you look inside to discover what works uniquely for you.

3. *Making lasting changes is hard work.* It requires a great deal of time, effort, commitment, and thought. Again: *It is hard*

work. Changing your life to this degree takes courage. Don't underestimate the amount of dedication and work required to make real changes. There are no quick fixes.

4. *You can do it*. You already possess all the strength and tools needed to succeed. Believe deeply in your ability to make the changes you seek. Victory over burnout starts in your mind and results in actions. You are in control.

I'm going to take an in-depth look now at several strategies you can use to prevent burnout if you aren't there yet and to heal from burnout if you've already crossed the line.

- ◄ Focusing inward

- ◄ Saying *yes* to saying *no*

- ◄ Learning to let go

- ◄ Getting support and feedback

- ◄ Exercising

- ◄ Paying attention to your diet

- ◄ Remembering to breathe

- ◄ Meditating

- ◄ Journaling

Focusing Inward

Pratayahara is a Hindu word used in yoga that means to draw your awareness *away* from the outside world and to refocus your attention on your inner being. It means to withdraw from the distracting sensory input of your eyes, ears, nose, and other sensory organs and quietly observe your inner self.

Learning to look inward is something everyone can benefit from, whether you're burning out or not. Most people spend so much time focused on what goes on outside them that they fail to tune in to what is happening in their own heads and hearts. It's easy to become drawn away from seeking out your own self.

This is equally true of finding your own way through burnout. Everyone burns out in her own way. Each person has a unique history and is affected differently by similar stressors; each of us heals differently. So it is a serious mistake to think there is one answer to recovering from burnout that works for everyone. I am repeatedly asked, "What can I do to get over my burnout?" Understandably, caregivers want simple answers and quick relief—everyone is looking for a magic bullet that can cure all ills. Because contemporary life moves so swiftly and we have become accustomed to multitasking, instant gratification, and speedy fixes for every problem, you're likely to be disappointed when you discover that making things better requires extended time and effort.

In a society overrun by drive-through outlets for food, coffee, booze, prescription drugs, and even weddings; in a society abounding in cell phones, instant messaging, shopping from the comfort of your couch, and video on demand, you shouldn't be surprised to find yourself expecting almost every whim to be satisfied immediately. It should also come as no surprise that you've grown so out of touch with your inner life. So to make any real progress—and that includes not reproaching yourself for your slow progress—you have to step back from all the worldly demands on your life and look inside for your answers.

Question: "What can I do to get over my burnout?"

Answer: "Focus inward."

The inner voice I mentioned earlier is constantly crying out for you to slow down and listen. It's probably so weary by now from trying to get your attention that it can't manage much more than a whisper. You have to settle yourself, focus inward, and listen attentively for that voice. What you will eventually hear is your personal truth; what you will see is your path beyond burnout.

As you read through the following suggestions for action, try one or two techniques that spark your interest. Not everything will appeal to you or be helpful to your specific situation. All of these tools and techniques can help you calm your mind and promote your happiness. Even so, no one-size-fits-all quick fix lies out there, waiting for you; only you will recognize the right answers for you—and most of them lie within.

Saying Yes to Saying No

In the introduction to this book, I reeled off a typical list of the things caregivers automatically say *yes* to. It's time to add something to that list: "Can you start saying *no* more often?" *Yes!*

When you finally start focusing inward and listening to that little voice, you will probably hear it saying that you are doing too much and that you need to say *no* more frequently. Saying *yes* to requests for your time, talents, and energy may seem to make everybody else happy, but doing so can deplete your reserve of energy and leave you feeling empty. Live like this too long and you're not going to be able to make anyone happy. Saying *yes* to some requests—those that you can fulfill without sacrificing your own mental and physical well-being—is rewarding. Agreeing to every request, however, is not only daunting—it's pretty much impossible. Yet far too many of you attended the "Say *Yes* to Everything" School of Living when you were young, and there you were taught a number of self-obliterating lessons:

1. *Don't make waves.* Most of us were raised to make other people happy and not to upset anyone. That means we were raised to say *yes* more than we say *no.* Saying *no* to requests rocks the boat and might make someone else mad or unhappy.

2. *Be socially subservient.* As I've noted, providers are often viewed by others, even the parents who hire them, as unskilled service workers or glorified babysitters, and they often take on that sense of not being important enough to disagree or refuse to do something, even when it's unreasonable. You can add to that the fact that the vast majority

of providers are women and that even now, in the early twenty-first century, much of society still views women as subservient to men. In some quarters, saying *yes* is almost expected when the request comes from a male in a position of power.

3. *Do anything to be liked.* You already know that you want to make people happy, and that if everyone around you is happy and well cared for, they will like you. You don't want to be thought of as defiant, self-centered, stubborn, or obstinate. You learned early that saying *yes* makes you a valued, important part of the group. And since you want to feel that the people who are part of your life truly value and like you, you say *yes*, even if *no* would be the more honest and healthy response.

4. *Take the easy way.* In most situations, it is simply easier to answer a request with a *yes* than a *no*. You want to be considered a team player. Saying *no* may mean disappointing someone or hurting her feelings, and then you may need to explain why you didn't say *yes*. Saying *no* may mean a confrontation. You conclude that the additional work and stress that come with some *yeses* are easier than the awkward or more complicated moment that comes after a *no*.

5. Yes *shows you're capable and strong.* Many people feel the need to show the world how strong and capable they are. That means saying *yes* to every new challenge, taking every opportunity to rise to the occasion—even when it means being run into the ground. Plenty of caregivers out there constantly say *yes* because they believe that saying *no* looks weak. The reality is that saying *yes* all the time shows greater weakness: you are powerless to stand up for your own needs.

Now, I'm not advocating that you go to the other extreme and start saying *no* to everything. That would be just as impractical and self-defeating as saying *yes* to every request. You need to find a comfortable, individualized middle ground. It is important that you feel free to make either choice, depending on your personal inclination, abilities, and needs, free of undue outside pressure. Here you can learn a lot from two-year-olds, who quickly figure out what a powerful word *no* can be and are unafraid to use it. Keep listening to that inner voice and empower yourself with a few well-placed, well-thought-out *nos* in your life.

Learning to Let Go

Learning to let go of stress is as important as learning to say *no*. Both are very empowering. When you hold on to the stress in your life, you give it unnecessary power. Holding on to stress also gives power to the people who are stressing you out. Back in my days as a center director, the decisions that unknown superiors used to make about my programs drove me crazy with stress. People hundreds of miles away and more concerned with statistics and dollar signs than services and people were making the big decisions. Their edicts often determined what I could and could not do in my program. Over the years, I held on to every bit of stress that their decisions stirred up. At times, the stress I felt while awaiting a decision about a new program or activity we wanted permission to start made me physically ill. It had total control over my mood, mind, and attitude.

Burnout is as much the product of your inability or unwillingness to let go of accumulated stress as it is of the external stressors you encounter. You internalize anger, frustration, guilt, fear, anxiety, and every other bit of negative energy you feel until you are ready to burst. And while you can't always change the stressors in your environment, you *can* change how much you hold on to them and the feelings they cause. I used to bottle up all the stuff that rubbed me the wrong way and unleash it on traffic, the weather, slow checkout lines, newspaper editorials, my dog, loved ones, and perfect strangers. I didn't know how to let things go, and even if I had, I probably would have chosen not to, just to spite myself. At some level, I believe I actually thought, "Why let something go when it's so much fun to feel miserable?"

If you are going to have any success getting past your burnout, you have to find healthy ways to let go of the pent-up emotional poison you're carrying. People and situations that upset you do not deserve that kind of control or that kind of power. I wish I could gain back the hours and days I wasted being teed off at people, things, and situations during my first thirty-three years. I could have done so much with that wasted time if I had learned how to let go of stress and anxiety.

Getting Support and Feedback

In an e-mail message to me, Cheryl, a child care provider from Nebraska, wrote, "My closest and dearest friends are the ones that I have made in my local support group. They just *get* me. We are all there for each other and know what to say for the good and bad days of our job. We laugh and have fun and look forward to our two times a month that we make a point of getting together. Once is for our monthly in-service meeting and the other on a social level doing things we like to do like scrapbook, go out for drinks, a movie, etc. Having at least 3 good friends that you can count on to be there for you and spend time with you having fun, is SO IMPORTANT."

Cheryl is right: some things about working as a provider can only be fully understood by other providers. Having understanding professional peers helps keep you centered. In *Secure Relationships*, Alice Honig observed, "You can respond with maturity and calm only when you are in tune with your own feelings. Tired, stressed-out caregivers need a friend or sympathetic coworker to whom they can voice their difficult emotions. When you feel a sense of loss after a child in your group moves to another setting, turn to a trusted adult to discuss your feelings. Sharing feelings lightens stress and helps prevent teacher burnout."

To deal with stress effectively over the long haul, you must become involved with some sort of peer support group. This can be an informal group that meets now and then or a more organized, professional association. National professional organizations exist to help you get involved with and feel connected to your peers. Here are my favorites:

◄ National Association for Family Child Care (NAFCC, www.nafcc.org)

◄ National Association for the Education of Young Children (NAEYC, www.naeyc.org)

For family child care providers' business needs:

◄ Redleaf National Institute (www.redleafinstitute.org)

If you are not affiliated with one of these organizations, I strongly suggest that you check them out and consider joining at least one. Both the NAFCC and the NAEYC have affiliated groups in many communities across the country. Many local providers' support groups and professional organizations eagerly welcome new members too. If you live in an area without a local group, consider looking to the Internet for support. Many online forums, chat rooms, and other resources are available. If all else fails, start reading the child care want ads in your own town. Find another provider in your area, call him up, and start a conversation. Chances are the person you called could use some peer support too.

Physical and professional isolation can become big problems for providers. Sometimes you feel as if you're always alone with the kids and never have contact with adults who understand you and your profession. Making the effort to build connections with your peers is a great way to reduce stress. You quickly discover that lots of other people share the same problems, frustrations, anxiety, and stressors. You also find people with similar hobbies, pastimes, passions, and senses of humor.

Collecting feedback about yourself is another way to reduce your isolation and connect with others. Feedback can be both educational— and scary. If you walk up to someone you know and ask, "Hey, how am

I doing?" or "What do you think of me?" you need to be fully prepared for her answer. If I had been brave enough during the year leading up to my burnout to ask Tasha for feedback, I don't believe I would have taken her answer well. It would have been good for me to hear her tell me I had turned into someone she didn't recognize or like, but I never thought to ask—and I doubt I would have accepted her reply.

Hilarie Owen, the author of *Creating Top Flight Teams*, has written, "Feedback is not always easy, and requires assertive communication and response. In other words, the feedback must not be a personal attack, but factual and accepted with agreement on what can be done to improve performance." Seek out someone you trust to give you honest responses to your request for feedback. Here are some possible sources of good feedback:

1. *Family members*. Your spouse and children are good sources of feedback on how you handle stress. Are you bringing it home? Have they noticed a change in your personality? Do they feel you have grown distant?

2. *Coworkers*. Asking for feedback from coworkers can cause anxiety, but it's one of the only ways you're going to find out if your stress is having an impact on your work.

3. *Peers*. If you are close to other child care professionals, consider asking them for feedback. They are removed from your immediate workplace, but they understand you and your job. It might be easier to ask someone you don't see on a daily basis.

4. *Children*. Children are very perceptive, so older children in your program can be a good source of feedback. Direct questions might be difficult for them to answer, but you can glean a lot about what they think of you and your performance through regular, honest, and open conversations.

5. *Program parents*. Seeking feedback from the parents you work for is a great idea. Start a conversation, tell them that

you value their feedback, and tell them you would like to hear how they feel about your relationship with them and their child and if they have any concerns. Listen attentively, and thank them for their candor.

6. *Your pet.* The feedback you get from Frito or Mittens may not be unbiased, but sometimes it feels good to chat with someone who won't ruin the conversation by talking back. Every question will be greeted with unconditional love, especially if you're scratching their ears and feeding them treats at the same time. If everyone else's feedback leaves you feeling down, ask your cat, dog, fish, or frog.

When you seek feedback, steel yourself for the worst and hope for the best. Take the feedback you're given and do something good with it. If you find that everyone around you believes that you are displaying the signs of burnout, take some action. If they say you seem fine, or happier and lighter than ever, keep doing whatever you are doing. Feedback is worthless unless you act on it.

Exercising

Putting your body in motion is a great way to fight burnout. Blood surges, sweat drips, fresh oxygen flows, muscles warm and become pliant, and endorphins (the neurotransmitters in your brain that act like morphine to reduce pain and give pleasure) increase. All these things change the way you look at the world. Whether it's from runner's high or yoga's calm, exercise does good things for your mind and body. The problem with starting an exercise program is basic physics: overcoming inertia. Objects in motion tend to stay in motion, and objects at rest tend to stay at rest. Getting into motion requires the exertion of force: you need to force yourself out of bed a few minutes early, force yourself off the couch, force yourself to put one foot in front of the other.

Once you have exercised your mind enough to start making changes in your life, I hope that a regular personal exercise program becomes part of your daily routine. All kinds of physical activities can help control your burnout. You may need to dabble a bit before you find the fitness program that works in your life, but it will be worth the search.

I want to share the exercise stories of two of my favorite child care professionals, Michelle and Shanna. Michelle has been working out regularly for a long time, and Shanna has only recently committed herself to regular exercise.

Michelle

Michelle walks. You can see her zipping along in the rain, in the dead of winter, in the heat of summer, early in the morning, and after dark. I went out at 5:30 one weekend morning in search of chocolate chip muffins and a newspaper; I barely had enough energy to drive. You can't imagine how lazy and out of shape I felt when I saw her striding along wearing a bright pink windbreaker and a huge smile on her face. I could barely choke down my two muffins when I got home.

Michelle's personal goal is to walk forty miles a week, 95 percent of them outside, no matter what the weather is like. In the past five years, she has logged over 9,000 miles. She tries to walk early so that she doesn't feel as if she is taking time away from her family, even when this means getting out the door as early as 4:30 in the morning sometimes. She lays out her gear the night before so she can wake up and go. "I don't give myself a chance to decide whether I want to go for a walk or not," she says. It has simply become another part of her life. Besides being great exercise, Michelle's walking routine gives her time inside her own head to think and sort things out. In a letter to me on the topic, she shared the following:

"When I feel stressed I go for a walk; and the minute the children leave I go for a walk. The clear air clears my head and gets me ready to face the day. It is exhilarating in any weather. When I walk I pray (for patience and understanding), I plan (my day), and

I plot (make lists and set goals). "After getting on a program, now in my 40s I feel better than I did in my 30s. Things started falling into place."

Michelle's walking has contributed to lower weight, a healthier diet, other exercise, a return to school, growing confidence, and greater feelings of self-fulfillment. She has that radiant, youthful glow that comes with health and inner calm.

You may be thinking, "Good for Michelle, but there is no way I could get myself out of bed that early and walk 9,000 miles in a five-year period." That's fine: you don't have to do what Michelle has done. You just have to focus inward and find something that can give you the same confidence and glow. Something that makes you smile and feel fulfilled.

Shanna

Shanna is a rural family child care provider. She lives with her husband and teenage son a few miles outside a small town in the Midwest. She started working out in the local high school gym, walking on the treadmill. In the first year, she went from wearing a size 16 to a size 12, and she says that now the 12s are getting loose.

Shanna's goal is to fit into a size 8 in the next few years. She has made working out part of her life. It hasn't always been easy, but she has repeatedly rearranged her schedule to make sure she can spend time in the gym regularly. Shanna has moved beyond the treadmill and now incorporates strength training into her workouts. She has lost weight, toned her body, increased her lung capacity, sped up her metabolism, and changed her diet.

The biggest change, however, has been in Shanna's attitude. She talks about the changes she has made as "habits for life." She says she has "a new outlook on life and lots of added confidence." I've known Shanna for a number of years, and she has always been beautiful, but the confidence she is so proud of is new. It casts a warm glow around her, especially when she talks about how she has managed to re-create herself.

You, Too, Can Be Like Michelle and Shanna

Michelle and Shanna have been successful with their workout programs, so they are repeatedly asked by others for tips and advice. Having others notice how their hard work has paid off makes them even more confident and recommits them to their workouts. I think they would both agree that it feels good to feel so good and that if they can do it, anyone can.

Of course, it takes some effort to get over your initial fear and inertia. Here are some tips to help you safely start your own exercise program.

- ▲ If you have not been exercising regularly, consult a physician before beginning your program.

- ▲ Pay attention to your body. Be mindful of aches, pains, and old injuries. Start slowly. It took you a long time to get out of shape; you shouldn't rush in to a new exercise program thinking you're as fit and limber as you may have been twenty years ago.

- ▲ Ease into your program a little at a time. Challenge yourself with small, achievable goals. If you set small goals and achieve them, you will build a history of success and that will build confidence. Success will help keep you in motion.

- ▲ Try to get at least a little exercise every day. When you are beginning an exercise program, the hardest part is breaking your old habit of not exercising. You need to set that habit aside and build a new one. In the beginning, taking a day off from exercise can make it very easy to take five days off—or maybe five weeks. When you're just getting started, consider making exercise a daily part of your routine. Small amounts of exercise every day help build up your exercise habit.

◄ Change your routine so you don't get bored. Michelle changes the route she walks, alters her speed, and makes other changes. Your exercise program should become habitual but not boring.

Once you have gotten yourself in motion, a whole new world opens to you. One of the benefits Shanna reaped from her program is flexibility, not only in her body but in her life. She is better able to bend and change as life requires it. I want that same flexibility for you; everyone needs to be able to stand firm and strong when needed and bend and twist when flexibility is called for.

Paying Attention to Your Diet

Food is such a major part of our lives that the way we interact with it can have a huge impact on us. Start by taking a closer look at what, when, how, and why you eat. Decide for yourself what changes you need to make. If you believe that changing your diet can contribute to a healthier you, go about altering it slowly, steadily, and thoughtfully. Don't make huge changes overnight; doing so will only add more stress to your life. Think, and then act mindfully. Are you eating because you're hungry or because you're seeking comfort? Do you stop eating when you're full? Do you eat a balanced diet with all the vitamins and minerals your body needs?

Both Michelle and Shanna reported that their exercise programs led them to eat more healthily. My experience has been the same. Once I started putting more thought into my actions and paying more attention to how I felt, I quickly realized that some foods made me feel energetic and others left me feeling lethargic. Over the past three or four years, I have been tinkering with my diet; in 2004, I woke up one morning and decided I was going to become a vegetarian. I didn't make this change for any ethical or philosophical reasons. For me, it was just the right bodily choice: I feel healthier, lighter, and more energized since making the change. Sometimes it isn't easy for me to choose an apple over an apple pie or a salad over a slab of ribs, but I've gotten to the point where I am making more good choices than bad. This is what works for me; you have to do what works for you.

Remembering to Breathe

Once in a while I get the chance to work with beginning yoga students. They are so focused on remembering which way to bend and stretch that they often have to be reminded to breathe. They start concentrating so hard on holding an asana (a yogic posture or way of sitting) that they forget the most basic part of life: *breathe in . . . breathe out.* Their faces redden, and they become dizzy. I release them from the pose, and they gasp for breath. In trying to do everything else right, they forget the basics.

Providers spend lots of time running around gasping for breath too. You get so busy with life that you forget to take time to breathe. Your body and mind hurtle from one stressful situation to the next. The world closes in. Your body tenses. Your chest tightens. Your stomach churns; you feel like Nemo on a six-day vacation in the Serengeti. If you're like most people, you hold your breath through the most stressful times in your life, depriving your body of oxygen at the time when you are most in need of it.

When you do remember to breathe, chances are that you don't do it very well. Most people fail to take advantage of their lungs' full capacity and instead breathe in short, shallow, quick breaths. This kind of breathing keeps you going, but deep, slow, long breaths do the job better, especially when you are in stressful situations. Making time to breathe creates a kind of temporal space in your life. It provides room to think, to organize thoughts, to calm frazzled nerves, to react mindfully. Whether you're kissing, singing, bow-hunting, jogging, speaking in front of a group, driving in heavy traffic, or working with children, your breathing plays a part in how well you do what you are doing.

After you've understood the following exercise, stop reading and give it a try:

1. Sit up straight. Lift your torso out of your hips and pull your shoulders back.

2. Close your eyes.

3. Inhale deeply through your nose.

4. Hold your breath for a second or two, and then exhale fully through your mouth, blowing out every bit of air from your lungs.

5. Pause for a second or two and repeat. Breathe in. Pause. Breathe out. Pause.

6. Again, breathe in through your nose. Pause. Out through your mouth. Pause.

7. Repeat this process six or seven more times.

This is important. If you didn't stop reading long enough to take a few breaths, do it now. This is something you shouldn't skip over; this is a simple but vital tool for dealing with burnout.

How do you feel? After nine or ten deep, cleansing breaths, most people feel calmer, more relaxed, and better able to focus on the task at hand. With a few breaths, you have managed to fully oxygenate your body, create space between you and your troubles, and tune in to your inner self.

Continuously breathing this deeply and mindfully as you go about your day may be difficult, but if you put your mind to it, you can slowly reprogram your brain to do it. Make it a point to think about how you are breathing from time to time during the day. If your breathing is shallow, take the time for a few deep, slow, long cleansing breaths. When stressful situations come up, breathe through them with those same deep, slow, long cleansing breaths. Afterward, think about how your slow breathing affected your behavior in the tough situation. I've found that better breathing never fails to help me handle unsettling situations more mindfully.

Meditating

In his book *Taking Responsibility: Self-Reliance and the Accountable Life*, Nathaniel Branden wrote, "We can choose to focus our mind, and we can choose not to. It is a choice we are constantly obliged to make. No other choice is more fateful for the kind of life we create for ourselves."

I learned to focus my mind from a great teacher who spends his days as an elementary school custodian. Chris Blades has been teaching Tae Kwon Do for around three decades. He has taught my daughter, and hundreds of other kids, to live the five tenets of Tae Kwon Do: courtesy, integrity, perseverance, self-control, and indomitable spirit. He doesn't just teach these tenets: he lives them.

A number of years ago, Chris started teaching yoga as well. He is the most naturally gifted, disciplined, in-tune, student-focused teacher I have ever met. He committed himself to focusing his mind, acquiring deep and wide knowledge of meditation and yoga, cutting through façades, and getting to the core of what his students need. These are what made him a good teacher. Chris had been teaching my daughter Tae Kwon Do for a few years when I decided I also could benefit from the class. At that time I was still consciously unaware of my own burnout, but looking back, I can see that my inner voice was pushing me to make a change. A few weeks after I joined the Tae Kwon Do class, Chris began teaching yoga, and I signed up for that class too. At the end of my first yoga class, Chris told me, "Let go." He had seen that I needed to relax, give up some control, and become looser. His words should have warned me that I was approaching burnout, but it took another year and a half before I hit bottom and quit my job.

I spent months becoming comfortable with meditating. At first, I could not sit still for two minutes without fidgeting; I felt nothing that could be described as *relaxed*. Over time, however, I began to catch occasional, millisecond-long glimpses of calm when I sat quietly and looked inside my hurried head. After plenty of steady, mindful practice, I have made meditating a habitual part of every day. It calms me, helps me to focus and make better decisions, and shapes me into an easier-to-live-with person. Looking back, I believe that learning to meditate and to let go, as Chris suggested, were instrumental in cracking the tough shell that years of internalized anxiety and stress had hardened around my soul. They were my first tiny steps toward freedom from burnout. I owe Chris a huge debt of gratitude; if I had not learned to meditate, I know deep in my heart that I would never have been able to focus my mind enough to write this or my first book, *Do-It-Yourself Early Learning*. Meditating has changed my life more than I can fully understand.

Meditating is a powerful tool for changing your mind. It's possible that you already have an informal meditation practice and don't even know it. Pausing to reflect at the beginning of your day; spending time alone inside your head while you shower, fold laundry, wash dishes, or enjoy a sunset; letting the calm of a morning run or an evening walk sweep over you; mentally rehashing your day as you drift off to sleep: all of these activities are examples of informal meditation. Learning to meditate more formally is at once the easiest and the most difficult stress-reduction skill you can acquire. It is easy because you can do it in any setting, in any position, without special equipment or clothing. You do not need to be physically fit or athletic. All you have to do is sit comfortably, breathe naturally, relax, and let your mind focus.

At the same time, meditating is one of the most difficult things to learn. That's because one goal common to most forms of meditation is to bring your awareness to rest in the present moment. Your mind is constantly flying from past to future to present and flitting from one thought to another thought. During formal meditation, you discover that your mind doesn't *want* to be focused; it wants to retain its customary, constant motion. This is called *monkey mind,* and it possesses us all. Think of your consciousness as a monkey and your mind as an endless forest. Your monkey is constantly leaping from tree to tree and from thought to thought. When you try to focus your mind in the present moment, thoughts drift in. Your monkey jumps to the "Did I pay the phone bill?" branch, hops from there to the "What's for dinner?" branch, leaps to the "My neck is sore!" tree, scampers down to the "Does my butt look big in these pants?" branch, and on and on. The more you try to control the monkey, the friskier he becomes. Rather than try to control him, simply acknowledge where he is, relax, focus inward, and let go. In meditation, your goal is to allow the monkey to still himself, to get him to rest for a moment in the present. One of the best ways to settle monkey mind is to observe with disinterest as he leaps from bough to bough. Eventually, his leaps will slow and he will settle himself in the calm of the present moment.

(While I was writing this page, I stopped to watch a squirrel climb a cottonwood, listened to Canada geese honk their triumphant return to Iowa, ate an orange, stoked the fire, and wondered what would happen if a squirrel and a goose got in a fight over an orange.) To be successful at meditating, you have to realize that you can't really *make* yourself focus; instead, you must learn to *let* yourself focus. The more you force yourself to focus, the more your mind resists. If instead you sit, breathe, and relax, without trying to force it, eventually your conscious mind will settle. Your "monkey" will pause in the present for a second or two. With practice, those seconds of calm will turn into minutes, and you will be on your way to meet the social and emotional risks and demands that accompany new learning.

GIVE MEDITATION A TRY: THREE TECHNIQUES

As a beginner, all you need to do is get comfortable, close your eyes, and relax. Here are some very basic meditation instructions for three simple techniques. They'll get you started.

Following Your Breath

—Sit, stand, or lie comfortably with your spine straight and your eyes closed.
—Breathe comfortably through your nose. Let your body relax, and allow tension to slip away from your muscles.
—Feel the sensation of your breath as it flows in and out of your nostrils. Feel the rise and fall of your abdomen or chest.

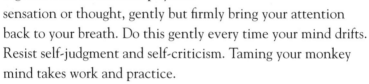

—Experience the beginning, middle, and end of every in-breath, and the beginning, middle, and end of every out-breath. Don't try to control your breathing, simply breathe. Let the breath breathe itself.

—Be aware of each breath as it enters and exits.

—Every time your attention wanders away from your breathing and shifts to another physical sensation or thought, gently but firmly bring your attention back to your breath. Do this gently every time your mind drifts. Resist self-judgment and self-criticism. Taming your monkey mind takes work and practice.

—Continue in this manner until the end of the time you set aside for this practice. (Maybe five minutes at first, working your way up to thirty minutes a sitting, or even an hour when you have time.)

—Slowly open your eyes, and enjoy the personal calm you have created in your busy life.

Visualization

Visualization is a different kind of meditation technique to bring calm and focus into your life. The goal of visualization is to transport yourself mentally to a different and more positive time, place, or reality. It may sound goofy, but it is a tool used by professional athletes and others to help reach their goals. Does visualization work? Well, I used to imagine being an author and living in a large old house full of kids. At the time, I didn't know what I would write, where the house would be, or whom the children would belong to. I even remember sketching the house and its many rooms. Over years of burnout, I lost track of this dream, but as I healed, the images popped back into my head. I revisited that dream frequently, visualizing more and more detail, until I was able to make this vision a reality: this is my second book, and I now live in a beautiful one-hundred-year-old–plus house that is filled each day with the laughs and joyous sounds of children in our family child care program.

Like following your breathing, you can use visualization anyplace, anytime. Before you get started, take a moment to decide what to visualize:

—If you want to relax, you may want to visualize a tropical beach at sunset, a suite in a swanky European hotel, a trip to a trendy spa, or a campsite in a lush green forest.
—If you prefer goal-oriented visualization, you may want to imagine yourself back in school, acing all your classes, succeeding in a new dream job, accomplishing the goals you have set in the job you have, dancing on Broadway, or moving into a new home.
—If you're anxious, you may want to visualize the resolution of the situation causing your anxiety. Picture yourself bravely facing the situation head on; doing so helps you build the courage needed to fix the problem.
—If you are out of tune with a child, parent, family member, or coworker, consider visualizing yourself as that person. Get inside her skin; see the situation through her eyes. Draw on all you know about her and imagine why she acts, and reacts, the way she does. This may provide some helpful insight into your relationship and may allow you to better empathize with her.
—If you just want to get away from your own life, visualize yourself as a soaring eagle, a leaf on a tree in the middle of a huge forest, an alien visiting earth, or the last unicorn. Take your time to decide where you want to go. It's your mental vacation, so go anyplace and everyplace you want.

To get started, sit or lie down comfortably. Take a few deep, cleansing breaths to prepare your body and mind. Let go of the day's worries and stresses. Relax in the moment. Close your eyes. When you are comfortable, begin painting a picture on the inside of your eyelids. You have decided where you want to go, so now let your mind take you there. You need practice, the ability to relax, and willingness to let go for this to work. If spending time rattling around inside your imagination is foreign to you, you'll need time to become comfortable with this practice.

Start by imagining the basic setting and then add details. For example, if you're visualizing a tranquil trip to the beach, start with a mental picture of the shore, the ocean, and the horizon. Now add yourself, as you want to be, to the scene. Who is with you? Can you smell the saltiness of the water? How does the warm sand feel under your feet? How do the waves and the birds sound? Do you see surfers, quaint fishing boats from the local village, or maybe large schooners on the horizon? Add a drink to your hand. How does it taste? Do you like the coconut cup and the cute paper parasol served with it? Are you proud of the hard work you did to fit into *that* swimsuit? What happens next?

Spend as much time as you need to flesh out your visualizations. Revisit them often. Create still pictures or movies. Add detail as the fog lifts from your eyes. Toss in some comedy, romance, or mystery. Let your imagination out to play. Create the same scene over and over, or visualize something new each time you sit down and close your eyes.

This is a powerful tool for relaxation, and it can help you turn your goals into reality. Before you can accomplish anything, you must be able to picture success. Visualize yourself living your bliss without burnout. Imagine handling situations before they get out of hand. See your dreams clearly, so you can devise a firm plan for making them real.

Progressive Relaxation

Our third meditation technique, progressive relaxation, is a simple but splendid way to relax and center yourself. Best of all, it only takes a few minutes out of your day. It's a great way to wake up gently in the morning, reenergize during the day, or unwind before going to sleep. The idea is to relax your body in stages, one part at a time. Enough talk—let's try it.

—Start with your toes and work your way up your body. As you progress, focus your mind on the feeling in your muscles as you tense and relax them. Breathe easily, allow your mind to clear, and focus inward.

—To get started, lie comfortably on your back. Just lie there for a few seconds and breathe deeply. Clench your toes and feet as you push them away from you. Now, still clenched, pull your toes toward you and hold. After a few seconds, unclench your feet and wiggle your piggies.

—Tighten your calves and hold. Take a few breaths and release. Flex your thighs and hold. Feel the tension in your muscles. Let your breath guide you. Release when you feel the time is right.

—There is no delicate way to say this: scrunch your buttocks, pelvis, and hips. Breathe. When you feel it is time to move on, release. We're halfway through. The lower half of your body should feel stress-free and calm.

—Squeeze your hands into fists. Squeeze hard, tightening all the muscles in your fingers, hands, and wrists. Breathe. Relax your hands when you're ready.

—Fully constrict the muscles in your forearms. Breathe; release when you are ready to move on to the next step.

—Your core is next; pull your abdominals taut. Hold them this way for a while; you'll feel them start to burn. Relax all your other muscles. Breathe. Release your abs when ready to move on.

—Tighten your upper arms; flex your biceps and triceps. Breathe, then release when you're ready.

—Keeping your upper back on the floor, pull your shoulders up and in. Contract your chest muscles. Keep these muscles tight, and relax everything else. Breathe. Let go when you're ready.

—Constrict the muscles in your neck; hold your breath for this one. Release and move on at your own pace.

—Scrunch your face so it looks like a raisin. Hold. Now go the other way: widen your eye, flare your nostrils, open your mouth wide, and stick out your tongue. Hold. No one is watching. Take a moment, and alternate between these funny faces a few times.

—Roll your head from side to side. Breathe deeply. Focus on the calmness that flows through your body. Don't be in a rush. When you are ready, sit up slowly and return to your busy life, refreshed.

Try all three of these techniques and use the one (or ones) most effective for you. You might use all of them, depending on your situation or the time of day. For meditation to be most effective, it's best to pick a technique that feels comfortable and to practice it on a regular basis, ideally at the same time each day and every day. If you can't do it every day, do it as often as possible. Like exercise, meditation takes discipline and practice for you to start reaping its rewards.

Journaling

Our final action step requires only a notebook (or a nice cloth- or hardbound journal, if you prefer), a pen, and a few minutes at the end or beginning of your day. If you're more comfortable at a keyboard, then you can use your computer. Journaling—that is, taking the time to put your thoughts, feelings, and ideas down on paper—can be a great way to sort out experiences and to clear your mind. As such, it can also be a powerful tool for preventing and curing burnout.

In an e-mail, my buddy Cheryl wrote, "I journal every evening as a way to finish my day. I like to write about the happy things that I experienced that day and work through any trouble that needs some attention by putting it on paper. I set goals for the following day and end on a positive note." Writing down abstract ideas and real emotions gives them physicality. When you journal, everything that has been floating around in your head can be seen and touched in the "real" world. Adapted from John Robson's list of one hundred benefits of journaling, here are twenty-five of the dozens of ways that journaling can help you reduce stress and unlock the inner you.

TWENTY-FIVE BENEFITS OF JOURNALING

1. Holds thoughts still so they can be analyzed and integrated

2. Releases pent-up thoughts and emotions

3. Disentangles thoughts and feelings

4. Connects inner thinking to outer events

5. Recalls and reconstructs past events

6. Helps you see yourself as whole and connected

7. Reveals and tracks patterns and cycles

8. Reveals outward expression of yet unrealized inner impulses

9. Clarifies relationships between thoughts, feelings, and behavior

10. Allows you to be your own counselor

11. Reveals your options so you can make better decisions

12. Reveals different aspects of self

13. Helps you see yourself as an individual

14. Finds the missing pieces and the unsaid words

15. Helps rid you of the masks you wear

16. Plants seeds for future change and growth

17. Focuses and clarifies your desires and needs

18. Awakens imagination

19. Enhances self-expression

20. Enhances breakthroughs

21. Unfolds the writer in you

22. Awakens the inner voice

23. Enhances memory of events

24. Allows you to let go of the past

25. Captures family and personal story

Become a Toddler Again

As you take action and begin making the changes needed to move beyond burnout, I encourage you to cultivate the joy, equanimity, optimism, curiosity, fun-lovingness, confidence, inner peace, and humor of a healthy, well-cared-for one-year-old. Look at the world with the fresh eyes of a toddler, seeing every person, situation, and experience you encounter as an opportunity to learn. Like a toddler, you will undoubtedly stumble and fall while trying to make changes in your life. When this happens, do what kids do: vent your frustrations, get up, and try again. This is a process that takes oodles of time and effort. You'll trip a lot and make mistakes, but a few missteps aren't enough to ruin a lifelong journey.

If you still don't have any idea what you can do to better your situation, relax. In the next chapter, I'm going to look at ways to get your mind to a place where you can focus and relax enough to see what you need to do.

Spend some time now thinking about the seven questions I posed to you at the end of chapter 3, using the tools we've discussed in this chapter. Journal about what your Ultimate Purpose might be.

◄ Let go of any anger or frustration you may have toward the three people that cause you the most stress when you practice progressive relaxation techniques.

◄ Visualize your ideal work environment.

◄ Address any feelings of guilt or fear that these questions bring about.

REFERENCES

Branden, Nathaniel. 1997. *Taking Responsibility: Self-Reliance and the Accountable Life*. New York: Fireside.

Honig, Alice Sterling. 2002. *Secure Relationships: Nurturing Infant/Toddler Attachment in Early Care Settings*. Washington, DC: National Association for the Education of Young Children.

Owen, Hilarie. 1997. *Creating Top Flight Teams*. London: Kogan Page.

Robson, John. 2003. From appendix 1: 100 Benefits of Journaling in "Go Deeper . . . Reach Higher . . . Journaling for Self-Empowerment." Higher Awareness. www.journalingtools.com/journalmaster3.pdf. Reprinted with permission of John and Patrice Robson.

Wycoff, Joyce. 1995. *Transformation Thinking*. New York: Berkley Trade.

Time Out

More Action Tips from Providers

During the last few years, I've kept a list of things that providers do to reduce their personal stress. Some of these suggestions come up frequently; some have been mentioned only once. These are all great ideas you can use if they meet your own needs. What makes them great ideas is that they really work for people. What ties them together is the deep personal value that people place on them during their journeys toward self-renewal and self-care.

◄ Date nights. One provider plans monthly date nights with her husband as a way to stay connected. They don't let anything interfere with their plans for quiet time together.

◄ Achieve a personal goal (big or small). A very personal goal one provider shared was her dream of acing some tests. She was working full time, going to school part time, raising her family, and still determined to get a perfect score on her three finals for that term. She worked hard at achieving the goal the week before she shared her story at a conference. Her face glowed with pride as she told it. Setting and achieving your own goals is a great way to build your spirit. I've heard about lots of goals that providers have set and met. Here are a few of my other favorites:

◄ One provider wanted to be brave enough to sing a solo at church.

◄ One provider made it a weekly goal to find time to shave her legs.

◄ Another provider made it her goal to laugh and smile as much as possible each day.

▲ My favorite is the provider who started regular workouts a year before her daughter's wedding so that she could wear the dress she wanted without the backs of her upper arms "flapping around like turkey wings."

▲ Find time alone. I have heard this one again and again. Many providers seek out a few minutes alone every day to clear their heads. Whether you take a morning shower, a long walk along a quiet road, or a ride on a loud motorcycle, your alone time is a valuable tool in the fight against burnout. A number of caregivers have described this to me as their chance to get in touch with their inner self—a time to tune out the world and tune in to their own thoughts.

▲ Ask your spouse to come home at noon. Remember the family care provider I mentioned who convinced her husband that her life would improve dramatically if he came home on his lunch hour and spent twenty minutes with the children so she could eat and use the bathroom in peace? It did.

▲ Ask people to leave. I've heard from many providers that the best thing they ever did for their mental health was to ask people to leave their home. Some family child care providers terminate care for families that cause stress or they enact policies that require everyone to be out of their home by a certain time each afternoon. Others have strict but unwritten rules for when they want company so that friends know when they are welcome.

▲ Dance. We've already talked about how exercise is a great way to get your body and mind in shape. Dancing is probably one of the least painful ways to exercise. I've met providers who make line, swing, ballroom, salsa, tap, and other forms of dancing part of their personal self-care. They explain that dancing is good exercise, takes their minds off their jobs, and offers wonderful social benefits.

◄ Take a beverage break. This can be a hot cup of black coffee in the kitchen at 4:30 in the morning while you read the newspaper; a glass of wine on the deck with friends while the sun sets; or a warm, relaxing cup of tea at night while you read before bed. In each case, there's something to be said for stopping what you're doing and simply enjoying your beverage of choice.

◄ Gardening. I can't dance, but spending time working in my yard is bliss. Many other providers feel the same. It's a chance to get some exercise and fresh air, commune with nature, and think.

◄ Pamper your body. From what I have heard, some of the most popular ways providers relax involve new hair styles, getting nails done, massages, and having things waxed. They don't click for me, but if spa treatments calm your busy mind, go for it!

◄ Leave work at work. Some providers have shared their techniques for building mental partitions between work life and home life. They have learned that bringing work home in any form causes them stress, and they have become adept at separating the two. I was never able to pull it off, no matter how much I tried. I let the job consume me—which was one of the reasons I burned out.

◄ Get a mammogram. One provider I met had just received the results from the mammogram she had put off for "way too long." She had found a lump and was so scared and worried that she actually made herself sick. She finally did what needed doing and discovered that everything was okay. She made me promise that if I wrote about her experience, I would be sure to tell you that "facing up to fears is much healthier than letting them eat away at your insides." If there is something that needs doing that you are scared to do, do it—then move on with your life.

▲ Remember that the kids do go home. One provider told me that no matter how stressful her day becomes, she always remembers that the children eventually go home—and not with her. This fact was very comforting and helped her make it through some very tough days.

▲ Enjoy a vacation, trip, weekend retreat, or day off. Caregivers work too hard and relax too little. Make time in your life for some rest, relaxation, and fun away from your profession. Doing so will recharge you and make you better at the job when you return.

5

Working with Whatever the Day Brings

Do a thing at its time, and peace follows it.

—Mandinka tribal proverb

EVERY DAY WE TRY to create safe, comfortable, and healthy environments that allow children to meet the social and emotional risks and demands that accompany new learning. Children, like the rest of us, need to move beyond fear in order to take the next step in development. They generally take such risks in stride—first brave steps, writing their name for the first time, making new friends, and exploring the world. Young children exult in the novelty of each fresh experience. For them, every new act or activity is a leap of faith, a step into the unknown. We cannot rush their learning, and we cannot do the work for them. All we can do is construct warm, inviting, loving, patient, safe, open, healthy places where they can face fears, risk failure, and progress at their own pace.

Creating stimulating environments is an important part of building a quality early care program, but doing the same for adults is not often thought of, particularly when it comes to providers' self-care. Like children, adults can only grow by facing fears and taking risks—preferably in safe, nurturing atmospheres. You need to create environments in which you feel secure before you can discard old ways of thinking and let go of old habits. If you want to change your life and move beyond burnout, you have to become proactive about creating such environments. Too many people simply wait and hope that things will change. They think life will magically become better when summer is over, when a particular child leaves their program, when they get their tax-refund check, when they start a new job, when they get their degree, or when a winning lottery ticket miraculously appears in their mailbox.

Deep down, most people know better. You know that if you simply wait for things to change, you're likely to be waiting a very long time. Improving your life requires thoughtful action on your part.

But I've Always Done It This Way!

All too often, people lock themselves into rigid ways of working and living. They look at situations with tunnel vision and fail to see the big picture. They look for quick fixes instead of seeking long-term solutions. They fall back on the same old failed strategies because they fear trying something new. Eventually, what were at first tools for dealing with life become a prison instead. If you keep using them, you become unable to see new ways of approaching people and situations.

In short, you become too set in your ways. Let me give you a simple example. For all of my life so far, my putting-on-shoes ritual has gone like this: left sock, right sock, left shoe, right shoe, tie left shoe, tie right shoe. That's the way my parents did it, and that is what I learned. That is how I grew up. It is what I know. It's the same with Tasha: left sock, right sock, left shoe, right shoe, tie left shoe, tie right shoe. We are left sock, right sock, left shoe, right shoe, tie left shoe, tie right shoe people.

Occasionally, just for fun, I like to mix things up a bit. I make sure that Tasha is watching—it's hard to irritate people if they don't see you do it—and I'll vary the comfortable routine like this: left sock, left shoe, tie left shoe, right sock, right shoe, tie right shoe. Diverging from my habitual way of putting on my shoes and socks feels physically weird, but seeing Tasha squirm makes it worth the discomfort. Witnessing such blasphemy—one foot completely clad and ready to walk out the door and the other utterly naked, with wiggling toes— drives her crazy. "Don't do that. It's not right!" she yells, turning her head away from my mismatched feet.

Life tosses people and situations at us, and mostly we react to them out of habit, using the rules we've created for living our lives. The majority of people are extremely good at living by those rules—so good that they fail to see other options. The problem with these learned actions and reactions is that they may lead you down the road to burnout if a new situation demands different responses. You can become bogged down in your traditional responses, not recognizing that other tactics, other choices and responses, are available. In his book *Rules for Radicals*, Saul Alinsky observed, "Tactics means doing what you can with what you have. Tactics are those consciously deliberate acts by which human beings live with each other and deal with the world around them. In the world of give and take, tactics is the art of how to take and how to give."

Providers need new tactics, more tools, and better strategies for dealing with the things that pop up during their days. Renae, a South Dakota caregiver who has found herself stuck in the snow physically and figuratively during her years as a provider, explained it this way: "Visualize how tires spin on ice—the engine is working and working and working, but the vehicle is not moving at all. If you can't change strategy (for example, rocking the vehicle, putting sand under the tires, waiting for spring), not only is the car STILL not moving forward, but you are wearing out the engine as well. Now you are stuck in the same place with a car that needs lots of repairs." She added, "The more I know, the more tools I have in my toolbox for the new and challenging situations that arise."

You should follow Renae's advice and fill your toolbox with as much helpful gear as possible. The more tools you acquire for dealing with situations and people, the more options you'll have for handling stressful and trying situations. But you need to actually use those tools; the better and more varied your tactics become, the better off you will be.

Your Own Personal Toolbox

You can't simply add tools without first shifting how you think about using them. You don't want to use only your grandfather's or grandmother's tools; times have changed, and perhaps they aren't as useful for today's tasks as newer ones. Too often, people allow situations to receive the same responses they've used in the past because they worked well in a similar situation twenty years ago. Why mess with something that worked?

You've acquired the tools in your kit from peers, parents, family members, teachers, friends, coworkers, public people you admire, professors, movie stars, authors, and even complete strangers. Sometimes these prompt what you do, and sometimes they prompt what you don't do. For example, I don't smoke because my dad did. I am a terrible speller because of bad experiences and lots of drilling from my third-grade teacher. Because of that same teacher, and lots of drilling, I know how to find the four directions and almost never get lost. I love working in my yard because it connects me to one set of grandparents, who farmed. I live in a big old house because it is where my other set of grandparents and my parents lived. I work with children because my parents were foster and adoptive parents, and my mother used to do family child care. I try to eat and live healthily because my family's history is full of heart problems. I don't drink too often and have never been drunk because when I was seventeen, I fell in love with a girl whose father is alcoholic. I learned to be outgoing and fun-loving because of a guy named Steve; before I met him in elementary school, I was too shy, introspective, and nerdy for my own good.

I became an adult the moment my son, Tyler, was born. I learned about loyalty from Sunshine, a German shepherd I owned in middle school. I learned the feel of heartbreak, and heartbreaking, from Tami, Patti, Corrina, Tina, a number of Jennifers, Tonya, and a few others. I learn about true love, commitment, interdependence, and friendship from Tasha every day.

These tools, forged from both personal and social history, helped form who I became and how I am able to react to life. When you learn to see your tools in that light, they can be put down and picked up as needed. The danger lies in believing that they alone constitute who you are and who you can be. Carrying around these tools can mask one of life's most essential truths: everything you need to be happy, to live your Ultimate Purpose, is already inside you. To get at your personal truths, you may need to put down some of the tools—for example, certain prejudices and bad habits, or certain fears—and instead focus inward until you can find new ones that are more effective in dealing with your stressful environment. You need to keep your toolbox organized: take care of the tools that work, get rid of the ones that don't, and always be on the lookout for new tools that may help do a better job.

A Tactical Manual for Burnout Prevention

In the previous chapter, I pointed out tools that you can use to start looking inside your mind and soul. Now let's look at some tactics you can use to deal more effectively with your daily environment; get closer to your inner truth; and throw away some of those old, rusty tools. These are the tactics I'll discuss:

- ◀ Make breathing space
- ◀ Develop situational empathy and concerned detachment
- ◀ Anticipate trouble
- ◀ Seek win-win solutions
- ◀ Cultivate a capacity for forgiveness
- ◀ Develop outside interests
- ◀ Stay flexible and keep your program fresh
- ◀ Grow professionally
- ◀ Be open and honest

Make Breathing Space

You can have so many responsibilities pushing and pulling you that you feel suffocated by your job. You may want to swoop in and fix things the instant you are able to identify the need for action, the second you can recognize that constant feeling of pressure, that sense that life is closing in on you and limiting your thinking, options, and control.

Wait a minute! While it's true that some issues may genuinely require instant attention, most do not. In fact, most problems can be better handled after you've given yourself breathing space and time for thought. Too often, people turn situations into emergencies just so that *something* gets done. They ask for your attention *now*, because for them, whatever issue they are dealing with seems as if the future of the world depends on its immediate resolution. Fortunately, this is rarely the case; in almost all situations, at least a little breathing room can be made. Even in the movies, the hero sometimes pauses to take a deep breath before attacking the alien spacecraft or defusing the bomb that's about to blow up.

When the situation allows, avoid rushing in with rash responses to questions or lightning-fast solutions to problems. Take time to form your solutions. Take time to breathe and think. Better yet, give things a chance to work themselves out before you venture in. Many problems, if left to run their course, resolve themselves or can be resolved by the main players without your involvement. For example, when children and coworkers are having a disagreement, they should be left to work out their own problems whenever possible. Solving their own difficulties empowers them and frees you for other things.

The stress of burnout often increases our tendency to rush from here to there to the next place, creating even more stress, when what we really need to do is slow down and create sufficient space in which to reflect and think. The act of stepping back is very empowering and gives you more control over your environment. Step back, and remember: *Breathe*.

Develop Situational Empathy and Concerned Detachment

Caregivers are empathetic people; it's what makes you good at your job. You can usually tune in to the feelings of the people around you with little effort. You feel what the children in your care, and their parents, feel; your heart and soul pulses in sympathy with their emotions.

So what's the problem?

The problem is that you can't really feel other people's emotions for them, and if you try to, the experience can be incredibly draining. If you absorb their troubles, successes, failures, hopes, dreams, anxiety, stress, and all the rest, your head becomes clogged with their emotional residue. You can't even be sure what you're soaking up is really theirs—maybe it's only your own projections.

To help keep your head clearer, try stepping back a few paces from overly close emotional ties with those around you. Instead, practice what is referred to as *situational empathy*. This means that instead of trying to *feel* other people's emotions, you instead *empathize* with their situation. You want to develop a clear, honest understanding of the situations in which children, parents, coworkers, and family members find themselves as well as recognize and affirm their emotions. When you can do this instead of trying to feel their emotions yourself, you can better maintain the genuine emotional ties you want. You are actually better equipped to help them when they need you too.

Practicing concerned detachment is another way you can protect yourself from becoming engulfed in other people's emotions. Sometimes in this profession you experience things that you would rather not see and learn things you would rather not know. I have had fourteen-year-old girls tell me they are pregnant because they were too scared to face their families alone. I have seen babies living in such filth that bottles sent home freshly washed the night before dripped baby roaches from the nipple rings when we went to mix formula the next morning. I've had to track down missing parents in trashy bars and drug houses when they failed to pick up their children on time. I've seen too many children's families disintegrate over problems with sex, money, perceived wrongs, abuse, jealousy, and every other thing that could go wrong.

When people you work with and care about are going through really tough times, you can empathize with them about their painful situations, but you also need to distance yourself mentally from their pain. I am *not* saying that you shouldn't be concerned and that you shouldn't do what needs to be done. What I *am* saying is that there are times when you need to detach from other people's lives and look at them from a more clinical perspective. Some of the situations I mentioned just now ate up pieces of my soul as long as I allowed myself to remain tangled in them. I allowed myself to be drawn in too deeply, and I invested too much of myself. Over time, I learned to detach, lovingly.

Such fond detachment is a hard skill to learn, but it is imperative, especially if you regularly encounter traumatic circumstances, as so many providers do. Writing about this topic, the burnout researcher Christina Maslach has observed, "The provider is genuinely concerned about people's well-being but has some psychological distance from their problems. There is neither too much involvement nor too little." It is important for you to find the balance that works. Maslach sees this balance as the "ideal blend of compassion and objectivity."

Anticipate Trouble

You know how Spider-Man can sense impending problems and react just in time to avoid catastrophe? Well, you can learn to develop your own "Spidy-Sense." Interestingly, as we grow more and more in tune with ourselves and become better at focusing inward, we also become increasingly skilled at tuning in to the people around us. By knowing what we feel inside, we can sort out our fears, emotional baggage, bad habits, and pain. Doing so frees us up to listen and observe others with a kind of sixth sense, an ability to anticipate problems and face them before molehills become mountains. If instead we are too wrapped up in our own unrecognized and unresolved issues, we're unable to deal with other people's troubles while they're still small and manageable. Life becomes a series of huge ongoing battles that could have been avoided.

Nothing magical is happening here—no superpowers have been created from a radioactive spider bite. It's really quite simple: when you get tuned in to yourself, you become more observant and better at notic-ing social cues, reading body language, and processing sensory input. You simply become more aware of your own and other people's signals, information that was always there but that you often overlooked or ignored. This skill makes it easier to differentiate the subtleties in an infant's verbalizations, decode the meaning behind the gleam in a pre-schooler's eyes, and interpret the body language of both children and their parents.

Like so many of the tools in your new toolbox, this ability to as-sess and react to people and situations more accurately gives you new power. You'll be able to head off problems before they get out of hand, and doing so will make life much more pleasant for everyone.

Seek Win-Win Solutions

In this competitive world, it's all too easy to think only in terms of winning or losing. You want to destroy your opponents and leave them quivering on the ground, sucking their thumbs. You want to win every argument, prevail in and dominate every exchange. Some of you are thinking, "That's not a problem in child care; most providers are women, and women don't act like that."

Well, when women are faced with the emotional overload that burnout brings, yes, they do. They may be socialized to play down their killer instinct, they may be better at hiding it, but when enough stress is present, it comes out. I've witnessed mothers and female coaches almost come to blows with female referees over calls in fourth-grade girls' volleyball matches. I've seen otherwise friendly center directors out for blood in battles over grant money. I've seen loving providers spew spiteful venom at parents during disagreements about the care of a child. And I've seen loving mommies spit venom back—all of this while the child looks on.

Such competitiveness only further alienates and isolates people, adding to your stress. When you feel the impulse building to top someone else, you need to practice your Make Breathing Space and

Concerned Detachment tactics and look for solutions that allow both parties to walk away winners instead of trying to defeat the other person. You can't tear down someone else without destroying a little of yourself in the process. Creating win-win solutions takes work, but with practice you can find ways to build equitable, just solutions in most situations.

Cultivate a Capacity for Forgiveness

To move beyond burnout, you have to build the capacity to truly forgive people for perceived missteps and misdeeds. I speak from personal experience: I have carried around resentments, irritations, and rage toward other people for years—with and without cause. And you know what? At the time, I enjoyed these feelings. I felt good, energized, overflowing with righteous indignation. I know I'm not the only one; at times, it seems as if being teed off and feeling slighted is the national pastime. The news is filled with stories of angry people suing, libeling, and stabbing people who they feel wronged them. Many politicians seem more like feuding toddlers than the political leaders our country needs.

Feeling hostility and enmity toward others uses up emotional energy that could be better applied. Why ruin your day being upset for the sake of being upset?

Of course everyone wants to hold tightly to his beliefs and personal truth. Eventually, though, for your own good, you need to let go of grudges and bad feelings—and it isn't easy. It's easy to *say* you have forgiven someone, but truly feeling and *acting* that way often takes work. Becoming strong enough to let anger and other bad feelings go takes a lot of personal growth and new focus, but the rewards can be huge.

Four- and five-year-olds are the best models for the kind of letting go I encourage. One minute they can be mortal enemies, fighting to the death over a toy car, and five minutes later they are happily eating snacks together, their epic battle already forgotten. Forgive and forget. Your life becomes much easier when you don't need to remember all the people you're mad at, and why.

Develop Outside Interests

The children whom providers work with are constantly learning and acquiring new skills; you should be too. Sometimes it seems as if all there is to life as a caregiver is the work. Providers are consumed by their jobs. Everywhere you go, the commitment to the children you care for follows you. At the grocery store, you see something they might like for a snack; at the bookstore, you stop by the children's section, although what you came in for was a trashy romance novel. Even on vacation, you can't resist the urge to drag back postcards, pinecones, and shiny rocks to show the children.

Not too long ago, I was in California doing some training. My son, Tyler, and his buddy Matt made the trip with me, and we spent some time at Huntington Beach. The boys were off being teenagers, and I walked along the shore picking up shells to bring back to our center to share with the children. After awhile, I stopped my shell

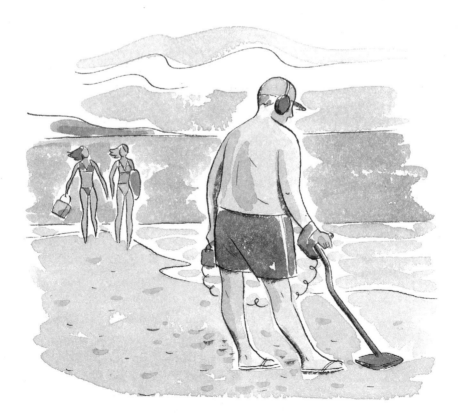

hunt and noticed that I had covered a lot of beach—beach covered with attractive women in swimsuits, whom I hadn't even noticed. I quickly realized two things: I had chosen a profession that it is hard to get away from. And I am officially old. The day I started focusing on shells instead of scantily clad women at the beach was the day I might as well have purchased a metal detector and started wearing my pants six inches below my armpits.

It's just good mental health, no matter what your work is, to have interests outside of your job. As a caregiver, you need to pursue kid-free interests, which may mean focusing inward and rediscovering parts of yourself that you've too often ignored and left to wither. Developing outside interests not only gives you something you can retreat to when your professional life feels burdensome; the creativity and self-esteem that come with exploring new parts of yourself also make you better at your job. Take a few minutes to think about what you want to learn more about, what hobbies you might want to pursue. As for me, I'm going to take a break from writing and search the Internet for metal detectors and old-man pants.

Stay Flexible and Keep Your Program Fresh

Some providers tend to cling to well-worn policies, practices, and philosophies long after those have ceased to serve their purpose. I have met kindergarten teachers proud that they did not make major changes to their classroom curriculum over decades-long careers. Proud that, even though the entire world changed dramatically over the years, their teaching methods and syllabus remained the same. Sticking to your beliefs and holding on to your values have their merits, but failing to flex and bend with the times can hurt the children in your care.

The world we live in today is drastically different from the world of fifty, or even five, years ago. Social mores, technology, family structures, and early learning theory have changed and evolved. As early care and education professionals, you need to change and evolve right along with them. Part of your duty is to stay flexible and up-to-date with changes.

Staying current and flexible does not mean embracing every passing fad or abandoning programmatic continuity. Flitting from one curriculum to another with the changing of seasons is as dangerous as continuing to do things one way because that's the way they have always been done; as with everything else, you need to make thoughtful choices about what to change and what not to. Spontaneity and experimentation keep your job fresh and bring professional rewards—good antidotes to stress and burnout. The key to incorporating change is to believe that it has a good chance of improving the quality of the program you offer. If you think it does, try it out—and be flexible enough to make more changes when they're needed, even if it's to undo what you've already done.

Grow Professionally

You grow and stave off burnout not only by discovering interests outside of work and tinkering with your work structure but also by continuing to develop as a professional. If you are regularly seeking ways to improve your job performance, you are less likely to get bogged down in petty annoyances and more likely to have an effective toolbox of tactics to deploy when difficult situations arise.

Too many providers fall into ruts where their professional growth is concerned. They cling to old ways of doing things and fail to seek new challenges, learn new strategies, develop new skills, and overcome old hang-ups. Growing professionally means different things to different people. Some of you may choose to return to school, others may opt for broadening your knowledge of early childhood topics, and others may prefer to deepen your mastery of a particular skill or practice. Let your inner voice guide your decisions. I've known providers who have expanded their knowledge of topics such as American Sign Language, Down syndrome, or separation anxiety because a specific child they worked with turned them down that road.

You always have something new to learn, something more to discover, in the profession of early care and education. The more you know, the more flexibility and control you have over your career. The demand for skilled and experienced caregivers is growing, and the wider and deeper your knowledge and personal experience, the more professional choices you will have.

Be Open and Honest

When you are filled with worry, fear, and stress, frank openness is a challenge, but as you learn to look inward for your own answers and grow more comfortable in your own skin, you begin to feel safer about opening up and sharing your ideas and feelings. The soil cracks open, and your new shoots seek the light and air, growing toward the sun.

As you come to know yourself better and overcome your personal fears, whatever they may be, you tend to become more open to new ideas and fresh perspectives. Letting down your defenses means you don't need to play all the mind games you previously used to protect yourself and to control situations. You become less manipulative and more willing to share your thoughts and feelings honestly. I used to fear sharing my real feelings and ideas because I worried that I would be judged harshly, that my every word would be dissected and picked apart. I feared looking dumb, sounding uninformed, seeming as if I was not in complete control of every situation. Now I freely admit that I am not the smartest person in every room. If I feel uninformed, I'll ask questions instead of trying to hide my ignorance. I don't need to look as if I'm in control of all situations, because I have better control of my own mind.

Being open and honest with the people around you can only lead to good things. It may not be easy, it may at times be downright scary, but it is much more productive and healthy than the games most people play with each other's minds. If you're driven by fear and defensiveness, relax—know yourself, and let others know you.

In the spirit of Honesty and Openness, I feel obliged to tell you that it's much easier for me to write about these strategies for working in a burnout-prone environment than it was to do the hard work that's made them part of my life. It takes trial and error, lots of focus, and a commitment of time and energy to internalize these strategies and make them your own. Don't rush these changes; make them mindfully. This isn't easy. Once you've made up your mind to change, your inclination is to jump in with both feet and try to fix all your problems at once. But you can't expect to make many changes at once without creating even more stress. Instead, make changes gradually and methodically.

I recommend that you select one of the tactics for preventing burnout from the list I've provided and then focus on living it as you go about your life for the next two weeks. Next, pick another and focus on *it* for a two-week period. Over time and with plenty of practice, these tactical tools will become second nature for you to use when you need them.

We've looked at tools like meditation and journaling that can focus your mind and clear your head, and we've looked at tactics like developing outside interests that you can use to deal with stressful environments. If you commit the time to use these tools and tactics mindfully, they can have a profound impact on reducing stress and preventing burnout.

In the next chapter, we're going to look at how you can move toward living your Ultimate Purpose, but first—homework. Go back again to the questions at the end of chapter 3. Review your answers to the first six questions and think about how the tools I've discussed so far can help you maximize the joy you get from your work.

REFERENCES

Alinsky, Saul D. 1989. *Rules for Radicals: A Pragmatic Primer for Realistic Radicals*. New York: Vintage Books.

Maslach, Christina. 2003. *Burnout: The Cost of Caring*. Cambridge, Mass.: Malor Books/ISHK.

Time Out

KIDZ Radio's **Caregiver Chat**

I've been talking to you pretty seriously for a while, so now let's stir things up a bit. I'm going to switch over to a great little pirate radio station I've been listening to for a few years and see what's on the air . . .

CHUCK: Hey, welcome back! You're listening to *Caregiver Chat* on KIDZ radio, FM 102.9. It's a sunny day, but from the calls we've been getting, it sounds like many of our listeners are feeling a bit cloudy and overcast. It's sad, but not unexpected, because today we're talking about the Big B . . . that's right—*BURRRRRRNOOOOOOOUT*. Lots of the lads and lasses listening right now are feeling out of sorts because the Big B and his ugly cousin STRESS have got them by the neck and won't let go. Let's go to Cindy on the East Coast. She says she feels like she's suffocating. Cindy—you're on the air! Take a deep breath and tell us what's on your mind.

CINDY: Hey, Chuck, thanks for taking my call. I work in a large center as the assistant director, and I, and I . . . excuse me, I'm a bit nervous. . . . I've never called a radio show before. . . . I feel like I'm drowning when I'm at work. There are so many people demanding my time, wanting answers and solutions, and needing me to do things for them and make snap decisions. I'm getting it from all directions. The staff, the kids, the parents, the director, the funders, human services— they all want something from me, and they want it five minutes ago. I don't know how much longer I can take it. . . .

CHUCK: Cindy, sounds like things are going pretty rough for you right now. Has this been going on long?

CINDY: I've been at this center for seven years, but the last year has been the worst. I was promoted to assistant director, and my life has been crazy ever since.

CHUCK: You've got a lot of people pulling at you. Can you share a few specific problems that we can try to address?

CINDY: Sure. My biggest problem is my director. She's wonderful, but she's stressed out, too, and she's always dumping stuff on me at the last minute. It drives me crazy. I don't mind the work, she just *always* waits until the last possible minute. The other thing that really stresses me out is that the staff members come to me with their problems and want me to fix them right away. Just the other day, out of the blue, Linda—she works in the toddler room—came to me and yelled that if I didn't get the carpets cleaned in her room by the next day, she was quitting. What should I do?

CHUCK: Cindy, it sounds like what you need is some breathing space. You're under a lot of pressure in your new position, and you've kind of let the walls close in on you. I think you should sit down with your director, tell her how you're feeling, and ask if she'll give you authority to make decisions about the tasks she routinely dumps on you. That way, you have more control over the timeline and don't end up feeling rushed and dumped on. It might even be a relief for her to hand over some tasks she dislikes anyway. Could you do that?

CINDY: It might work. We get along really well and she trusts me to do things; that's why I got promoted to assistant director. What about the other problem—got any advice?

CHUCK: Yes, I do. I think you should tell Linda that this is the first time you have heard a thing about her carpets needing cleaning and that you don't like being threatened. Let her know you'll look into it when you get a chance and that if the rugs do indeed need cleaning, you'll get it scheduled as soon as possible. And let her know that if this is something she wants to quit over, she has every right to make that choice. Be calm and matter-of-fact. This allows you to step back from her threat without escalating things. If she doesn't quit—and I doubt she will—ask her to talk to you *before* she feels a situation has become so critical that she believes it's worth quitting her job over. We've got to move on, Cindy. Thanks for your call.

Patrice, you're on *Caregiver Chat*—what's happening?

PATRICE: Weeeell, Chuck, I'm a family child care provider in a rural western state, and I've got a problem with one of the families I provide care for. The kids are great, but the parents are going through a rough patch, and I must be the only one the mom can talk with. I hear about everything that is going on in her relationship. I don't want to go into too much detail, but there are some issues that really make me uncomfortable. There was an affair, there has been some violence . . . I hear about it all. Sometimes she shows up to pick up the kids and doesn't leave for an hour and a half. She makes herself comfortable and unloads all her emotional stuff. She cries so much that she sometimes gets me going, and by the time she leaves, I'm an emotional wreck. I want to be supportive and do what I can to help, but it's like I'm too close to the situation.

CHUCK: Patrice, I'm going to make a wild guess here. This isn't the first time this has happened to you, is it?

PATRICE: You're right. It seems like someone is always unloading all their emotional crap on my living room carpet. I'm not a therapist, but everyone seems to think I've got the answers to their problems.

CHUCK: You're not alone. This is a problem lots of providers have. As a group, we're really empathetic people. People with problems feel comfortable and safe talking to us. Apparently we exude care and concern from every pore, and people with problems can just sense it or something. Anyway, you have a couple of choices here. You can let things keep going the way they are, burn out, and be looking for a different job within the next three years. You can start kicking people out of your house when they start venting their personal problems, which probably isn't going to make you feel good, and it's likely to cause other problems for your business. Or you can work to change your own mind a little bit. You sound like you're allowing yourself to become overly involved in other people's powerful emotions. I want you to try empathizing with the situation this woman is in and not identifying with the emotions she is feeling. This will allow you to step back, keep your emotional equilibrium, and remain more objective about the situation.

PATRICE: So I'm supposed to just stop feeling? I'm supposed to listen to all this emotionally gut-wrenching stuff and not *feel* anything? That sounds easy, Chuck. I've watched *Titanic* eighteen times, and I still can't make it through the DVD without crying my eyes out. What the heck are you talking about?

CHUCK: I don't want you to stop feeling. I want you to feel for the situation that's *causing* her emotions rather than *feeling* her emotions. Feel sorry for the kids, feel sad that this relationship is falling apart, but do not allow yourself to become washed away by the emotional tidal wave she's bringing into your relationship. Empathize with her situation, not her emotions. It will take practice, but it will protect you a bit from all the strong emotional stuff you're bombarded with every day.

PATRICE: Okay, I think I see the difference, and I'll give it a try. You're right, though; this doesn't sound easy. Can't you give me a simple solution?

CHUCK: There aren't any simple answers. There's one pretty simple thing you can do, however: put an end to her hanging out and un-loading on you so often and for so long. Let her know you want to be there and be supportive, but that you can't have her hanging around that much because you have commitments to the children in your care and to your own family. Limiting the time she spends venting will also help you keep a clear head.

PATRICE: Thanks, Chuck. I'll give it a try.

CHUCK: Great! Call us back in a few weeks and let us know how things go. We're going to take a break now, but we'll be back in a few minutes with more listeners' calls. You're tuned to *Caregiver Chat* on 102.9.

ANNOUNCER: At the end of a long day of caring for other people's children, it's time for the Quiet Time Inn. We offer professional care-givers a child-free environment where they can get together and have some fun. This week all your favorite appetizers are on special, and we'll have a different blues band playing each weekend for the next month. If the kids have been loud all day, it's time for quiet time at the Quiet Time Inn, located right off I-64 between the airport and the Industrial Interchange. That's right, listeners—the Quiet Time Inn is a great place to get together, unwind, and relax.

CHUCK: Now, let's hear from Sarah. Sarah, you're on the air. What's happening?

SARAH: My life is like a rollercoaster, Chuck. One minute things are going great, and ten minutes later I'm in the dumps. I feel like my job as a child care provider has consumed me. I don't know if this is what I want to be doing with my life. I don't recognize myself when I look in the mirror. I don't know where I'm going. Any advice?

CHUCK: Sarah, you're struggling, and you're not the only one. Lots of providers come to points in their careers where they question whether they have followed the right path in life. I suggest you spend some time rattling around inside your own head and really think about who you are and what you want to be doing with your life. If you're not happy as a provider, it will soon begin to show in the quality of your work, if it hasn't already. Mindful introspection is what you need. Sometimes we get so busy with life that we forget who we are and where we wanted our lives to lead. If you don't feel like you're living your Ultimate Purpose, maybe it's time for a career change.

SARAH: I started working with kids because it was something I loved, but for the last few years, it just hasn't been that fulfilling. I've got some other interests I'd like to pursue, but frankly, I'm scared. I don't know if I'm up to the challenge.

CHUCK: Why don't you find a hunk of time and a quiet space and try to pull your thoughts and ideas together? Maybe get them down on paper so you can actually see what you've been thinking. Ask yourself some hard questions about your present and future. That may help organize things in your mind. Making changes is a scary proposition, but living a life you're not happy with is probably worse. You deserve to be happy, and if being a provider isn't doing that for you anymore, you owe it to yourself and the kids you work with to make a change. I can't give you any simple, magical answers, but I can tell you that you're not alone in feeling this way. Good luck and best wishes.

We're going to take a break for the business news with Herb Garden, and then we'll be back with more calls. Herb?

HERB: Today's story comes from CHILD-CON in Las Vegas, the annual convention featuring the latest in new high-tech child care equipment. An anonymous entrepreneur from Iowa has led a team of scientists working in a secret laboratory for several years to develop microscopic robots called *nanobots* for child care providers to use in their programs. He's given them names like Snot-Bot, Slobber-Bot, and Poo-Bot, because they scurry around, digesting all the gross stuff that oozes out of small children. Apparently they are self-replicating and convert what they eat into fuel. They're quite spendy—$15,000 for a starter set of seventy-five nanobots. Back to you, Chuck.

CHUCK: This guy from Iowa clearly has too much time on his hands, Herb. We have our last caller on the line, and she's from north of the border. Kelly in Winnipeg, you're on the air.

KELLY: Thanks for taking my call. I'm having a problem with the kids I care for, and I need some advice. They keep messing up the toys. I've set up lots of great learning areas: a block area, dress-up area, car area, manipulative area, and many more. The problem is that the kids keep moving the toys from one area to another, and by the end of the day, we have a big mess. I like things nice and tidy, and these children are anything but cooperative. What should I do?

CHUCK: Kelly, it's almost time for the news, but I think we can handle your situation before the break. It sounds like the children are doing exactly what their little minds and bodies were designed to do. They are playing, exploring, and discovering the world. They are making connections with materials and with ideas. Why does this bother you so much?

KELLY: I spent a lot of time setting up my classroom, and I want that to be respected. I'm giving them lots of materials and different activities to choose from, but they just go and do whatever they want. Yesterday they hauled all the baby-doll blankets clear across the room so they could use them to make tents in the block area.

CHUCK: It sounds like you've created a great environment that they find very engaging, and they're taking a lot of initiative and making creative use of the materials you've provided. Do you think it would be possible for you to be a bit more flexible when it comes to how they choose to use the materials? Sometimes kids have ideas for ways to use materials that we adults would never think of. Try to allow them more leeway in their play, but also make sure they do most of the picking up when the time comes. They need to be able to use the materials as they see fit, as long as they are being safe and respectful of your equipment and learn that the natural consequences of making a big mess is having to clean it up. Think you could give it a try?

KELLY: They do enjoy themselves, and they *are* learning. I suppose I can work on being more flexible, but it might take me a while to get used to the whole idea.

CHUCK: That's understandable. As adults, we need to be open

to change, but our minds get used to doing things one way, and it's often hard to change. Good luck, Kelly.

Thanks for listening, everyone! Tune in next week, when we'll be discussing vacation days and health insurance—or the lack of them. Keep fighting the good fight, and remember to breathe. We now return you to your regularly scheduled book.

Like so many other radio call-in programs, Chuck's show doesn't have the time to look really deeply at most issues. The fact is that no one tool will solve problems as complex as these callers'; it takes an entire box of tools that you've become comfortable using to make progress against burnout.

6

Seeking Your
Ultimate Purpose

"I BECAME A FAMILY child care provider in 1992, worked six years, and totally burned out on the long hours, lack of professional respect, and family stress resulting from the family child care business."

"I find myself, at least daily, questioning my career choice."

"These children are God's great gifts. I want to receive the gifts from these children they freely give each day: their unconditional love and their enthusiasm, joy, and curiosity. I love discovering what makes them tick. I love providing that teachable moment! I love the challenge of figuring out their needs and personalities, and seeking a better understanding of their behaviors."

As a parent, which of these providers would you want caring for your child? Which one sounds as if she is dealing well with stress and the other challenges that come with a career as a caregiver? Which one sounds as if she is on a path to her Ultimate Purpose?

These words are pulled from e-mails I've received from caregivers wanting to share their thoughts on the topic of this book. So many providers have shared stories of feeling bogged down, broken, drained, shattered, incomplete, tense, unfulfilled, empty, or deficient. These feelings of discontent run deep, permeating every corner of their lives both at work and at home. Everyone strives for fulfillment and happiness in work. The strategies and tools I've discussed in the previous chapters can help you examine your career choice and seek out your

Ultimate Purpose. If you do the hard work required, you can move from burnout to a life of fulfillment and new beginnings.

Of the three providers quoted above, Pam, who wrote the third passage, seems to be the only one on the road to her Ultimate Purpose. She and I have probably spent less than twenty minutes talking in person and have only exchanged a few e-mails, but her passion for her job shines in her every word. I'm sure her life has its ups and downs, but I know she is able to balance them. I have no doubt she is doing precisely what is right for her life right now.

A Wise Teacher Said ...

What could be better than that? What could be better than full engagement with your own life and a full commitment to mindful living?

Moving from burning out to seeking your Ultimate Purpose is a challenging task requiring courage and endurance, but the rewards can be amazing when you open yourself to a new world of opportunity and possibility. Getting past your burnout is difficult enough, but preventing it from sneaking back into your life can be even more daunting. Your new, healthy mind-set and outlook require constant upkeep.

Feed the Good Dog

I have committed myself to making yoga and meditation parts of my daily routine, but some days my practice is half-hearted. I have committed myself to a healthy vegetarian diet, but some days I eat more chips and chocolate than I should. I have committed myself to staying fresh and focused, but some moments are musty and blurry. I have committed myself to living in the here and now, but sometimes I drift into the past or dream of the future. I have committed myself to being fully in tune with the people who touch my life, but some of my interactions are completely discordant. I have bad moments, even days, but I always focus on feeding the good dog.

Here's a Native American story I heard about a tribal elder who was sitting near a blazing campfire with his grandson. The wise old man says, "I have two dogs that live inside me: a good dog and a bad dog. The bad dog always fights with the good dog."

After pondering this for a while, the youngster asks, "Which dog wins?"

The old man replies, "The one I feed the most is always victorious."

Life flows smoother when you make every effort to feed your good dog. The bad dog may still start fights, but the good dog always wins if he is well-fed. Feed your good dog.

I used to beat myself up about my momentary setbacks and struggles, but I have come to realize that I need to expect and accept bad times. Realizing that I'm not perfect and don't have to be was a freeing revelation. I try to make peace with the off moments of my day and focus on what went right. Teach yourself to be vigilant, and make self-renewal a part of every day. If you can do this, you open yourself to the prospect of living your Ultimate Purpose.

Do or Do Not

It's Friday evening. Three tired and stressed child care providers stroll into their favorite hangout, the Quiet Time Inn, after a long day of work. The bartender welcomes each by name while preparing their favorite drinks. Trading greetings with other providers as they cross the room, they settle into their much-loved corner booth. You've seen biker bars, cop bars, lawyer bars, and artist bars; this is a child care provider bar. No kids allowed; no color crayons, no diapers, no booster seats. (The Quiet Time Inn does, however, provide sippy cups for patrons who like to take their drinks onto the dance floor.)

The women order dinner and drinks as they take turns rehashing their week. They talk of kids, parents, policies, backaches, and biting, but, as usual, after twenty minutes, the conversation turns to other topics. They have work-related stuff to get off their chests, but they swear never to let it consume their whole night. Three years ago, when they started this weekly ritual, they agreed to vent over appetizers and then to shift the conversation to other topics.

Each week they speak eloquently of life and love. They hold deep and meaningful discussions about relationships, dreams, and passions. They share intimate secrets and deep desires. They mentor each other, supporting their efforts to realize dreams and desires. They nurture each other's bliss and galvanize each other's commitment to living their Ultimate Purpose. Frequently they reminisce about the night they first met, the unlikely night their little group formed.

Each of them had wandered into the Quiet Time Inn looking for a place to sulk, lick her wounds, and contemplate life after yet another stressful week. They had never met before, but the waitress said they looked as if they could be friends, and she seated them together in what would become "their" booth. A long, dark conversation, lasting through two bands and many margaritas, began. At the time there were five members in the group. Two of the five worked in centers, one "watched kids" at her house, one worked in a Head Start classroom, and the last taught in a church-based preschool. They were all running on empty and ready to quit their jobs. Words like *drifting, empty, unfulfilled, meaningless, fruitless, anxious, agitated, disconnected, confused, lost, unrewarding*, and *frustrating* peppered their conversation. They shared unmet dreams and desires. They spoke of paths not taken. They talked about feeling out of sync with their own lives, as if they existed in a time zone that was a second or two behind the rest of the world. They told of sleepless nights, queasy stomachs, and chronic headaches whenever they thought of work and of how hard it was to constantly "be there" physically and emotionally for kids and parents. They agreed that they needed to make changes, and they agreed that they probably would not do so—their shared misery was too enjoyable. They agreed to meet every week for a "bitch session."

This went on for a few months. They got together, grumbled about work and life in general over dinner and drinks, and went home feeling satisfied, wallowing in group melancholy.

Then one dark and stormy night, while the group was mid-bitch, the door to the Inn slowly opened and in walked Yoda and Kermit the Frog. The two vertically challenged green guys sauntered up to the unhappy providers and smiled congenially. Yoda pointed his wooden staff at them and said, "Frog says it not easy being green."

Without a pause, Kermit added, "Do or do not. There is no try. That's what my buddy the Jedi says." With that, the pair of green friends winked, bowed, tipped their top hats, ambled over to the bartender, and ordered two bottles of Moose Drool.

Stunned, the women began to discuss what had just happened. What in the world could the two vertically challenged sages have meant, and how did it relate to their predicament? Then a quiet man in white sneakers and a sweater joined their group. He sipped his cocoa and said, "Hello, neighbors, it's good to see you! I couldn't help overhearing what just went on, and here's what I think they meant. Some of the things life deals you are out of your control, like being green, but you have the power to make the best of them. You can change your environment, or the way you react to it. You can do it, or not. I think they meant that you have the freedom to change if you want to. You can live like you're living now, or you can live your bliss." With that, he finished his cocoa, left a very generous tip, and headed out the door.

The women sat stunned for a moment. But it wasn't long before they began talking all at once, each of them vowing to make changes that would alter her downhearted predicament and fulfill her Ultimate Purpose.

It took time, but slowly their lives began to change. The woman who "watched kids" in her home professionalized her family child care business and went back to school. One of the center workers began to write short stories in her spare time and eventually had one of her stories published in a national magazine. The Head Start teacher quit her job and started her own small child care center. The other two left their jobs to pursue dreams unrelated to children and child care. It wasn't easy, but with each other's support, all of them managed to make positive changes in their lives, thanks to the words of Yoda, Kermit, and the kindly stranger.

Lessons from the Green Guys

When Yoda said, "Do or do not. There is no try," he was declaring that there are two clear and basic choices in life. You can either:

1. Do

   OR

2. Do Not

Simple as that.
We can act OR not act.
Say yes OR say no.
Change OR live with the status quo.
Look over the next hill OR stay in the valley.
Fight the current OR go with the flow.
Speak up OR keep quiet.
Open the door to new experiences OR keep it tightly closed.
Turn on a light OR sit in the dark.
Gather information OR jump to conclusions.
Talk OR listen.
Be happy OR be discontented.
Choose paper OR plastic.
Make good decisions OR make bad decisions.
Find your Ultimate Purpose OR burn out.

The OR is what's important. It gives you a choice; you always have a choice. That choice may not be of what happens to you; it may be of what you can do with what you're given. In every situation, during every minute of every day, whether you think you do or not, you have choices. There is always an OR floating in front of your face. The problem is that you get so busy living in the past ("I wish I had told her what I really think") or the future ("I can't wait until the weekend") that you aren't able to live mindfully in the moment and to see the OR. You dwell in your past and dream of, or dread, your future. Meanwhile, the present slips by unnoticed. You do the same things, make the same mistakes, dream the same dreams, over and over again. You become stuck in a cycle of repeatedly wishing for change and then being paralyzed by the cynicism that is the hallmark of burnout.

Even with all the power they possess, some people cannot overcome their fear of change, so they put their dreams on hold and defer their bliss. Others either consciously or subconsciously choose to remain in a state of burnout. It becomes their unhappy, but perversely comfortable, norm.

Which brings me to Kermit's "It's not easy being green." Kermit and his greenness blend into the swamp. He doesn't stand out, he isn't flashy or sparkly—just green, like everything else in his world. He didn't choose to be green; it's just the way he is. A wise frog, Kermit realizes he has no control over his greenness and can't alter it—but he does have a choice: he can choose to learn to be comfortable in his own emerald skin OR to struggle against his greenness. He chooses to live with himself the way he is. In fact, he learns to look at his greenness as beautiful. From him, you can learn to love yourself the way you are, warts and all. You may not have control over your external circumstances, but you can always change your mind.

Questions from the Heart

A tribal proverb from the Omaha Nation says, "Ask questions from your heart, and you will be answered from the heart."

When you start looking at your life as a child care provider, you may find that it needs some adjusting to make it the career you want, or you may discover that child care is not what you want to do at all.

Too many child care providers simply fall into the profession. They start their caregiving career as a detour—something to do while their own kids are young, a way to make a few bucks until they get the job they really want, or a way to get work experience that pays a little while they're going to school. They have every intention to leave the field in a few years—after all, they started working with children with no aim of making it their life's work. Then they wake up one morning twenty years later and realize that they have let their real dreams slide beyond their grasp.

I've heard providers talk about feeling trapped in the wrong life. They headed in one direction and ended up someplace completely different. The life they currently live lacks something—some unfulfilled dream, some unmet desire. Some providers look deep inside their hearts and find their Ultimate Purpose nearby; others find they need to change careers to move toward the life they should be living.

Determining Your Purpose

When you start looking at your motivations, dreams, desires, hopes, and wants, you can't know what you will find. Be prepared. This isn't an easy task. Determining what you are truly here to do can be tough, and actually living it can seem impossible.

Here are the first steps: Carve time out of your day for yourself. Sit in a quiet room, close your eyes, take a few deep breaths, relax, and ask yourself the following questions:

   ◢ Am I REALLY happy OR am I putting up a front?

   ◢ Do I REALLY want to work in my current position OR do I want to do something else in early education?

   ◢ Do I REALLY want to continue to work with children at all OR do I want to work in another profession?

   ◢ What would make me feel more comfortable in my own skin?

   ◢ What makes my heart sing? What is my bliss?

◀ What dreams do I want to make real? What calls me?

◀ Where do I see myself in five or ten years?

◀ What is my Ultimate Purpose?

Your answers probably won't reveal themselves in a single sitting. Make time to meditate on the questions regularly. You can start by simply sitting and thinking. As time goes by, solid answers begin to form in your head; clear ideas emerge from the fog. You should not rush this process. You've probably spent many stressful and anxious years wandering away from your dreams; you shouldn't expect to recover them all at once. The better your idea of where your Ultimate Purpose lies, the better your chance of getting there.

As you dream of your Ultimate Purpose and set goals to reach it, remember that your dreams and goals do not have to be huge. I've asked a lot of providers what their goals and dreams are, and many burst out that they want to have a million dollars and live on the beach or that they want to be famous. These are fine dreams if they are heartfelt, but most of us have simpler dreams—ones that don't vary too much from the lives we are already living. These simpler dreams are just as valuable as the grander ones. What is important is that the dream is *yours*, that it reflects your own hopes and needs. Once you have recognized that a dream is really your own, set do-able goals that can make your dream a reality, and embark on your journey toward the Ultimate Purpose of *your* life.

Moving from Dream to Reality

Once you have a good idea of where you need to go, you have to do the hard work: moving from Thought to Deed, from Idea to Reality. Making your dreams real takes work. All sorts of methods for achieving goals exist, and many people are willing to sell you their programs for success. The following are techniques I use. I'm a child care provider, not a self-help guru, but I'm willing to share what is working in my life. In the end, you have to find the methods that work best for you. After you have some idea of what your Ultimate Purpose is, consider some of these suggestions for setting goals that can move you toward living the life you want.

◀ Set vivid goals

◀ Write down your goals

◀ Plan, plan, plan

◀ Identify hazards and sacrifices

◀ Build a timeline

◀ Talk about your goals and plans

◀ Make time for your goals

◀ Break down big goals

◀ Start with the small stuff

◀ Take the first step

◀ Take action daily

◀ Meditate on your goals

◀ Evaluate and update

Set Vivid Goals

When it comes to setting personal goals, the more detailed they are, the better. Taking the time to build a powerful vision for your life can have big payoffs, and the process of setting realistic goals helps bring your vision into the world of the achievable. Use all of your senses in building your goals. When you close your eyes, you should be able to see, hear, feel, smell, and taste your dreams. The clearer your vision of what you want to achieve, the more achievable it becomes. Infuse your goals with as much definition, form, and life as you possibly can.

This is where visualization, the meditation technique I described in chapter 4, comes in handy. Remember the beach scene in which I described visualizing the smell of the surf and the sounds of the beach? This is the technique you should use when visualizing your personal goals.

What is your goal? What does your face look like when it is finally achieved? What are you wearing? How do you celebrate? Who is with you? How do you feel? Do you have goose bumps? Are you smiling? How does success taste and smell? What colors do you see? What is the setting? What are you going to do next? Are you relieved your journey is over, or is this success just a step toward a bigger goal? Picture the smallest details of the goal you desire to bring to life. Invest your dreams and goals with vibrant emotional detail.

Vibrant dreaming not only makes your goal feel more real; it also gives you a clearer understanding of where you really want to go on your journey. This is *your* goal; you have to be completely honest with yourself while dreaming it. The more you visualize this goal, the more real it becomes. Because you are endowing it with so much reality, you should not be surprised if it takes on a life of its own and begins to evolve and change. Pay attention to these changes, because they may be your mind's way of telling you that your path needs adjusting or that your goal has changed.

Write Down Your Goals

Take the time to write down what you're thinking. Write, don't type. Taking the time to put your vivid goals and dreams down in your own handwriting is an investment. Putting your thoughts down on paper helps make them real; it transports them from the metaphysical world, the world of imagination, into the physical world. They also become much more difficult to ignore when they are staring up at you in your own handwriting.

The good news is that writing down goals is the first step toward encountering your own magnificence and living your Ultimate Purpose. The bad news is that you may believe your goals can't be reconciled very well with where you currently are in life. The life you want to live may be far removed from where you actually are. Such a realization may seem like bad news initially, but consider it a blessing: the differences between your reality and your goals can help you map out your journey and determine how to get from Here to There. Once you've written down your powerful goals, it's time to get to work on planning how to make them real.

Plan, Plan, Plan

You cannot plan too much when you are trying to achieve personal goals. Take the time to list the steps you need to take to get from where you are to where you want to be. Living your goals is serious work and should be thought of that way. It's as simple as this: if you don't plan, you won't achieve. You can have the clearest, most vivid goal imaginable, but if you do not invest time in planning how to achieve it, it won't happen.

Different people plan in different ways. Some people prefer to sit down at a desk and work with calendars and task lists, while others do all their planning in the confines of their head, only later jotting down notes on legal pads as their goals take shape. Others do a bit of both. It doesn't matter how you plan as long as you plan.

Identify Hazards and Sacrifices

The more pitfalls, hazards, roadblocks, U-turns, sacrifices, and other obstacles you can map out as you plan your journey toward your Ultimate Purpose, the easier the trip will be. Too often, people rush into new adventures without really mapping out their trips. They fail to educate themselves about what might hold them back, and then they feel surprised when reality steps in and slaps them in the face.

The hazards on your journey will be very personal. They may be conditions of the soil you're growing in—a personal mind-set or a hang-up that holds you back. They may be influential people in your life who, for whatever reason, want to block your progress. You may encounter financial barriers and limits on your time or energy. Whatever the hazards, they will be much easier to overcome if you anticipate their existence, prepare for them, and plan how to over-come them. Confronting these obstacles during your planning process may be frightening, but it's better to plan for them than to encounter them unexpectedly on your journey toward your goals.

Build a Timeline

Building a timeline gives your plan some structure and organizes the tasks you need to complete to move your goals from thought to reality. Arrange the steps you need to complete in a logical order and give each a completion date. You may be able to hold all of these steps in your head, but putting them down on paper probably makes it easier to visualize the work ahead. Think of your timeline as a map to your goals. You can build a very detailed timeline, with each and every step of the journey plotted out, or you can simply include major landmarks along the way.

Do not beat yourself up if you miss a deadline or find that you need to adjust your timeline. It's only a framework for you to work within, a way to provide some structure for your journey. If life gets in the way—and it will—adjust and update your timeline as needed.

Talk about Your Goals and Plans

Once you've set your goals and made your plans, put them out into the world. Talk to the people in your life about what you want to accomplish. This is another way to make the work that lies ahead feel real. Putting it out there also makes it harder for you to abandon your efforts when the going gets tough. If you talk up your plans, you are less likely to let them fall to the wayside, because no one likes to look as if he has failed or given up. Another benefit to talking about your goals and plans is that the people you talk with may share their ideas and insights. They may have valuable information or strategies to help you achieve your goals. Don't go overboard—you don't want to scare your friends and family away by constantly talking about your big plans and goals. You just need to make sure that the important people in your life know what is important to you. The ones who show special interest in your goal to live a more fulfilling life will make their interest known, and they will become your support team and cheerleaders.

Make Time for Your Goals

Life is distracting, and making time for your goals will take some effort. I'm writing this page during the kids' naptime on a beautiful July afternoon. Since many of my current goals are related to books I'm writing or want to write, I plan out some quiet time for writing each day. Even so, when I try to focus, I am repeatedly distracted by the breeze blowing through the trees outside the window, the sound of a train in the distance, the fish gliding through the aquarium in flashes of silver and orange, and the throaty rumbles of the toads in the terrarium a few feet away. I've made time to work on my goals, yet I still have a hard time getting the work done. If you don't plan time to work on your goals and then do the work, you won't experience any forward motion.

You have to learn to say *no* to distractions. It's not easy. Life will try to distract you. Relaxing in the sun, reading a good book, eating ice cream, and sitting around feeling sad that you're not living your dreams are ways you can spend your time, but such activities must be set aside now and then if you want to achieve your goals. Make time to do the work—and then do the work.

Break Down Big Goals

Question: How do you eat an elephant?

Answer: One bite at a time.

(Note: Please don't start eating elephants. They are endangered, they are great parents, and besides, I hear they are high in cholesterol and go straight to your hips.)

Achieving big dreams can look like a daunting task when you're at the beginning of your journey. You may be so overwhelmed by the amount of work lying ahead of you that you're reluctant to take that first step. Before you begin your journey toward your Ultimate Purpose, you should break your big goals down into smaller, easier-to-achieve ones. Breaking them into bite-size pieces makes them more manageable, and therefore more achievable.

Start with the Small Stuff

It's important that the first step you take to begin your journey is a successful one. So tackle the small stuff first. You broke down the big tasks; now start your journey with a few small, simple steps. If your goal is to earn a college degree, the first thing you might want to do is to arrange some study space in your home. If your goal is to run a marathon, your first step may be to acquire some new running shoes and socks. Give yourself a chance for success by first taking on tasks that are easily achievable. Doing this builds a history of success, bolsters your confidence, and moves you a few steps closer to your ultimate goal or goals. You have to start someplace, and the best place is usually with something small.

Take the First Step

It's time to get to work. Taking the first step toward your newly set goals is the hardest part of the journey. You need to break free from inertia and set your plans and ideas into motion. You have to move from idea to action. It's difficult to start down a fresh road when you have spent a long time sluggishly struggling only with the daily tasks of living. Understand that any reluctance you feel when taking your first step probably comes from some unresolved fear of the unknown or the new. It's hard to move in a new direction when you've grown comfortable with the status quo. Taking the first step toward your goals is all about overcoming your fear of change and leaving old habits behind. The easiest way to do this is just to plow through the fear and move from thought to action.

Take Action Daily

After you break free from inertia and take your first step, make it a habitual part of every day to work toward your goals at least a little.

Every step you take is a step closer to success. Working on your goals every day means that you are always making progress. A little work each day adds up to a lot of progress over time. Working on your plan should be as much a part of your daily routine as brushing your teeth or eating; make it one of those things you just do.

You do not have to accomplish something big every day. For example, if one of your goals is to organize and de-clutter your home, you may be feeling overwhelmed by the size of the job. Tackling the entire job in one weekend might be impossible, but a small amount of work each day makes the task manageable. If you work on it a bit at a time, spending only ten or fifteen minutes filing, sorting, or putting things in order, in the course of a few months you should have a much neater and more welcoming living space. As you train yourself to work daily toward your goal, you'll begin to notice successes and feel better able to tackle bigger and bigger pieces of your goal.

Meditate on Your Goals

I have touted meditation as a valuable tool for improving self-awareness, focusing the mind, finding inner peace, and harnessing the power of Self, so not surprisingly, I think meditation should also be used to turn your goals into realities. Meditating on your vivid goals and dreams is a powerful tool. Meditating etches your desires into your mind and helps focus your efforts. With practice, it helps you to clear out much of the muck and murk that clogs your thinking.

To meditate on a goal, sit comfortably, as I described in chapter 4, and begin to meditate. As you relax, bring the powerful image of your goal into your mind. Allow this image to permeate your being; breathe it in and out. Doing so brings you close to it, and you will find that answers to problems and ways around obstacles in your path simply appear.

If you are not experienced with meditating and still have not given it a try, this probably sounds silly, but here goes: Years ago, I would have agreed with you. Fortunately, experience is a wonderful teacher, and she has taught me that meditation is an unbelievably powerful tool for improving your life.

Evaluate and Update

Course corrections are a part of every journey. As you work through your plan and timeline for achieving your goals, make sure that you pause periodically to evaluate and update your plans. You undoubtedly will need to make changes as you move along. Taking time to evaluate your activities and make changes to your plans acquaints you with how far you have progressed and how far you still have to travel. Evaluating your efforts may reveal important information, provide insight into more effective ways to progress, or reveal that your planning has been top-notch. Such a review gives you realistic feedback on how your journey is progressing.

Some Final Thoughts for Your Journey

Working toward your Ultimate Purpose is a very personal endeavor. You must chart your own course and make your journey alone. Your travels may deepen your commitment and passion for early care and education, or they may lead you in entirely new directions. You are seeking a life in which you can be joyously optimistic about each new day, passionate about the tasks you undertake, serenely confident in your abilities, and eager for new challenges, so your journey will take a very different form from everyone else's. But the challenges you encounter in getting there and in maintaining your balance and equilibrium once you have achieved some success are similar to those of many other seekers. Here are some additional ideas that have helped me on my journey; they may be helpful on yours.

- ◀ Make it easy to succeed

- ◀ Know what you need to know

- ◀ Seek support along the way

- ◀ Open yourself to success and opportunities

- ◀ Fake it until you make it

◀ Change your mind if you need to

◀ Record your actions and successes

◀ Be firm but flexible

◀ Celebrate success

Make It Easy to Succeed

As you work toward your personal dreams, do everything you can
to make it easy to succeed, because you can make achieving success
simple or hard. Which is it for you? You may need to rearrange your
physical space, carve out special alone time in your day, purchase
special materials or equipment, or something else. Spend some time
thinking about your goals and how you work; you'll discover things
that can make your tasks easier.

Know What You Need to Know

From the beginning, you need to educate yourself about what you'll
need to know along your journey. Spend time determining what skills,
abilities, and proficiencies you need to develop to achieve your goals.
Invest time at the beginning of your journey to find out what you
don't know. To do this well, be open and honest with yourself. Don't
gloss over anything or try to trick yourself into believing that you
know more about something than you do. Personal honesty can save
you from embarrassing situations later on. Like me, you probably have
tried to fake it through certain situations by pretending to know more
than you do; don't let this tendency trip you up now. First figure out
what you need to know on your journey, and then start learning it.

Seek Support Along the Way

I've already written about the importance of getting the support
of colleagues, mentors, and friends as a way to buffer yourself

against stress. Doing so is equally important while you move along the path to realizing your Ultimate Purpose. Being out in the wilderness alone, headed for your Ultimate Purpose, is scary. The journey becomes much easier and more fulfilling if you have a solid support team. You're more likely to succeed if you surround yourself with experienced mentors, energetic cheerleaders, loyal friends, qualified teachers, and knowledgeable guides. The support of professional organizations like NAEYC and NAFCC can be valuable too.

When you head toward new places in your life, it's helpful to seek out people who have trod the path you are heading down, people who already know the lay of the land. Don't walk blindly into unknown territory when you can look to others who have been there for advice on the terrain. Let me give you an example. Eight months before the publication of my first book, I started to worry because I didn't know how to be an author. I didn't worry much, though, because I knew I would have many chances to observe seasoned early childhood authors at upcoming conferences. Since then, I've watched authors present to small and large groups, I've watched them at book signings, and I've sought their advice. I am slowly starting to feel comfortable as an author. What I learned from observing and talking with others has made the process easier and much less stressful than it could have been. Remember all those tools you've collected to help deal with your stress and burnout? Well, one of the best ways to learn how to utilize them in your life is by observing someone proficient in their use.

Your journey is your own, but you don't have to make it in solitude. You need a helpful group of supportive people on your journey to offer advice, celebrate successes, mourn setbacks, hone visions, and overcome obstacles.

Open Yourself to Success and Opportunities

Do you know people who always succeed, who live happy and fulfilled lives without doing any apparent work? It's as if the Success

Gnome and Happiness Fairy are following them 24/7, constantly sprinkling them with Magic Achievement Dust and carrying them over any rough patches that life tosses in their direction. At some point in your life, you have probably wished these lucky folks ill so that they could learn what it's like to live a normal life, like yours. You may be jealous of their apparent effortless success, but you can learn a lot from them.

The reality is that these people work hard and do not have mythical creatures helping them through their days. The big thing they do that most people don't is this: they freely invite success and opportunities into their lives. When you are open to good things happening, good things are more likely to happen. Too many people walk through life expecting the worst so that they won't be disappointed when it happens; what they need is to open themselves up to the good in life and come to expect success. As you deepen your inward focus, doing this becomes easier; at times, you may feel as if an unseen hand is guiding you through your day.

Fake It Until You Make It

Another thing you can learn from those people who walk around happy and successful all the time is to act as they do. You need to learn to fake it until you make it. If you look successful and happy, act successful and happy, and think as if you're successful and happy, eventually you're more likely *to become* successful and happy. You need to live your goals. Act like the person you want to be, even when you don't feel like that person.

Change Your Mind if You Need To

As with so much else in this book, finding your way down the path to your Ultimate Purpose involves bringing about mental as well as physical change in your life. You have to change from Someday thinking to Today thinking, from Try thinking to Do thinking, from I-Wish thinking to I-Can thinking. You have to continue to tune in to your essential self and then be honest with that revealed self.

Record Your Actions and Successes

I've mentioned the importance of writing down your goals and recording the successes you experience along the way. Doing so is important because recording your history will prove helpful if you need to question your progress or begin to feel bogged down. Besides, being able to look back on where you started and see all the work you have done will make your eventual success taste even sweeter.

Be Firm but Flexible

As you work to achieve your goals, remain firm in your commitment to the course you charted toward your Ultimate Purpose, but be flexible too. Life progresses, things change. Too rigid a mind-set can be harmful, because there are a lot of things you don't have control over that can influence or alter your plans. If you are flexible, you will be more prepared when life steps in and knocks you off course along your journey. Be firm, but be flexible.

Celebrate Success

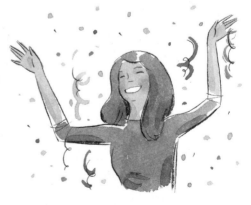

Never miss a chance to celebrate success along the route! The easiest way to keep moving toward your goal is to keep up your spirit, and the best way to do that is to celebrate your achievements. The type of celebration you choose is up to you. Some people have parties with lots of friends and family; others prefer smaller, more personal commemorations of their successes. Celebrate in your own way, but take the time to rejoice when you reach your milestones. Doing so gives you energy to keep on keeping on, and it reinforces your commitment to your dreams.

Smile at the Kids and Mean It

I hope that you have found some tools in these pages to better handle the stress innate to your profession, to overcome your fear of making changes and become more comfortable facing the unknown. My hope is that most of you who read this book will find your Ultimate Purpose within the profession of early care and education and that those of you who leave the field go on to a life of heartfelt joy and happiness.

If you feel that you simply cannot smile at the kids anymore, you need to make changes. You need to revitalize and refresh your passion for your career or find a new one. Life is too short to invest time and energy in work that leaves you unhappy and unfulfilled. You deserve happiness, and the children you work with deserve a caregiver who can effectively handle the downside of the profession. They deserve providers with *real* smiles.

I'll say this one more time: making the changes you need in your life will not be easy. Real change takes personal commitment, introspection, and constant work. You'll need to keep focusing inward, strive to peel away the accumulated layers of fear and bad habits, continue to care for yourself, and persist in seeking out your Ultimate Purpose.

I came very close to walking way from a profession I deeply love and losing much that I care about. I don't want this to happen to you. I want you to be able to do your job with all the passion, emotion, joy, love, forthrightness, humor, integrity, and glee it deserves. I want you to live a balanced life and to love your work again. I want you to live mindfully and feed the good dog. I want you to smile at the kids and mean it.

Appendix:
Tips for Directors and
Supervisors

BURNOUT CAN RUN THROUGH A CENTER like a virus, infecting staff members one after another. I've seen it happen firsthand, and I've been the recipient of many stories shared by providers during conferences and via e-mail. Remember, most burnout comes from the environments in which you operate, environments over which most providers do not have much control. Directors, other supervisory staff, and the providers they oversee commonly personalize their burnout, blaming themselves for their condition.

Burnout can be even more infectious when it starts at the top. If you as a director are running on empty, your feelings undoubtedly will trickle down to your staff. No matter how much you try to hide or ignore your burnout, it will be reflected in your program. You can't keep it secret (my experience is that you can't keep *anything* secret in a center), so you had better make dealing with your own burnout a high priority. Make time to take care of yourself so that you can effectively take care of your program.

"I plan as many get-away weekends as I can or that I can afford. I feel that the weekends help ease the burnout more than a week's vacation. It always gives me something to look forward to. And I try to plan at least one day off a month," says Pat from Massachusetts via e-mail. These are great tips for directors. You can't keep other people motivated, happy, energized, and on task if you're not able to be these things yourself. Most directors I know believe they have to be, or at least have to *appear*, perfect. They put on a strong face for staff and families, even when they are crumbling inwardly from all the stress. They are overworked, overextended, overtaxed, and overdone.

Let me give you a vivid example. When she was asked to share insights for this section, one director I have known for years replied that she had nothing to contribute because her program didn't have such problems. Her staff, however, saw things very differently. The staff members viewed her as angry, short-tempered, on edge, unwilling to confront problems, turning a blind eye to situations that needed attention, and ineffectual. They saw their program as on the verge of collapse, fractured, and struggling. The director loves her job and claims not to see any problems; her burnout has blinded and numbed her to what her staff sees, thereby paralyzing her ability to take action.

The saddest thing about this situation is that lots of you will read the above paragraph and think that I'm referring to *your* program. What it all comes down to is this: the best thing you can do for your staff and program is to take a clear look at yourself and deal with your own burnout. If you aren't feeling burned out and think things are peachy in your program, be brave enough to ask your staff members for their honest assessment of the situation—and be ready to deal with their responses.

Look closely, because even programs that seem perfect on the surface often have problems lurking in the shadows. I met with one group of caregivers during the California AEYC conference in Anaheim in 2006 who worked in a program that had resources most providers would love: full health benefits, paid vacation days, regular breaks, supplies, better-than-average pay, and a director whom staff genuinely liked and respected. As we sat in the excessively comfy lobby chairs of the hotel, these providers nonetheless vented frustrations with their program. A few of the employees, they told me, were infected with burnout: they didn't pull their own weight, they weren't reliable, they didn't interact well with the children. The group felt that the "problem staff" didn't fit into the center's program. Dealing with these people on a daily basis had the providers I spoke with ready to quit their better-than-average child care jobs and move to programs with worse benefits and better work environments.

Building a Provider-Friendly Environment

Once you've taken care of yourself, build an environment that is more provider-friendly. The resources and time necessary to implement the following suggestions vary, but anything you do to reduce stress among your center's employees is worth the investment. I'm going to explore some of the basics you can provide your employees with to build healthier center-based environments.

◀ Real relief (including regular breaks)

◀ Clear expectations and feedback

◀ Useful goals and training

◀ A voice in planning and decisions

◀ Productive meetings and planning time

◀ Professional relationships

◀ Competitive benefits

Real Relief

Over the past few years, I have talked with hundreds of providers who work in center-based programs, and what they most want to alleviate stress and prevent burnout is regular breaks. Working with children is physically and emotionally demanding, and to do it well, providers need time to clear their heads, take care of personal needs, and rest a while so that they can remain fully present for children. They need time to calm their minds and nerves. Too many providers are working eight hours or longer a day without a single real break. Five minutes to use the bathroom is not a break. Sitting with the kids during naptime is not a break. Running out for supplies is not a break. Making snacks is not a break.

Providing breaks is definitely a scheduling and budgetary challenge, but regular breaks lead to happier, more productive, less stressed staff. They also help reduce absenteeism, lateness, and turnover.

It doesn't have to be big, but regular action to offer real relief from stress is a great way to cut down on burnout in your program.

Clear Expectations and Feedback

In some programs, staff members walk around in a daze because they do not know what is expected of them. They were hired, tossed into a room full of kids, and left to sink or swim. They don't understand what their responsibilities are or what the heck they are supposed to do to keep their job and make the boss happy.

Life is better for everyone when you know what is expected of you. Tossing an unprepared caregiver into a room of children is potentially as dangerous as tossing a plugged-in toaster into a bathtub. Ensure that all staff members understand exactly what is expected of them while they are on the job. They cannot know these things unless you tell them. Here are some suggestions for clearly communicating your expectations:

- ◢ Make sure everyone working in the program knows the program's mission, goals, and philosophy.

- ◢ Create detailed job descriptions for each position.

- ◢ Develop a staff handbook and a policy-and-procedure manual detailing how situations should be handled. If you have these documents, make sure they are updated regularly and that what is in them matches the way the program actually runs. Then make sure each employee gets the handbook, reads it, and fully understands what it says.

◄ Hold regular staff meetings that are productive—that is, meetings that have clear goals, an agenda, and are efficiently run.

◄ Assign experienced mentors to new staff people so they have someone to go to when they encounter problems.

◄ Be certain that everyone understands the center's organizational chart. Employees need to know how information is supposed to flow, whom they report to, and who reports to them. It is vital that all staff members know where they fit in the larger scheme of things.

◄ Use clear and concise language when talking about expectations—and everything else. Don't be wishy-washy.

◄ Remember to express your appreciation when staff members fulfill your expectations. Write a heartfelt thank-you note for work well done. Send flowers or another small gift of appreciation at appropriate celebratory milestones. Hang a giant "thanks for all you do" banner for staff members to discover when they arrive at work.

◄ Encourage parents to share their appreciation and gratitude.

Unclear feedback is another problem that can contribute to low staff morale. I've heard over and over from center staff members that they receive mixed messages from their directors—things like: "You're really doing a wonderful job with the toddlers, but I wish you would spend more time outside and not be as messy during snacktime," or "I think it is wonderful how you are down on the floor keeping the infants so active and engaged, but you really need to keep the toys picked up better."

Be clear with your feedback to staff members—either they are doing a "wonderful job with the toddlers," or they need to spend more time outside and be less messy. Being down on the floor engaging the infants is most important, or keeping the toys picked up should be the primary focus—it can't be both. When you stick a big *but* in the middle of a sentence, remember that it tends to negate everything that came before it for the hearer. She walks away believing that your praise was hollow, only stuck in to make it easier for you to get to the meat of your complaint. If a staffer is really doing a wonderful job, tell her. Then shut up, smile, and walk away. If you have a complaint, share it in a forthcoming and unambiguous manner. Say what you mean and mean what you say. Using clear feedback will unmuddy the waters and lead to better communication between you and your staff.

Finally, giving providers positive feedback and rewards, including trust, for work well done is absolutely crucial. I cannot put it any more simply than this: if you truly do not trust the people working in your program, find new people to work for you. If you truly trust them, make sure they know it, and reinforce your conviction at every available opportunity. When you are ultimately responsible for the health, safety, and well-being of small children, you must really and fully trust the people in your program. I've know directors who were shackled to their centers with titanium cable because they did not trust their staff members enough to leave them alone. These directors didn't attend meetings, they didn't take breaks, and they didn't take vacations. They were in the center from open to close with an eagle eye locked on the staff. If someone isn't doing his job, give him clear feedback on how he must improve, and if he doesn't meet your expectations in a reasonable time, let him go and hire someone who can do the job appropriately. Once you have a team that you fully trust, give its members more rewards, responsibility, autonomy, and freedom to act. This will prove to them that they are trusted and empower them to emerge as leaders. Your trust also means that you can turn your eagle eyes to other tasks and maybe relax a bit yourself.

Useful Goals and Training

All staff and directors should develop a list of long- and short-term goals, personal and professional. When burnout takes over, most people go on autopilot, losing track of dreams, ambitions, and bliss. Putting down your goals in writing creates a target and a reference point that you can go back to when your will is flagging. You must know your destination before you can map your course. My burnout blew me off the path to my goals for many years. It took a long time to get on track again. Spend some time helping your staff members develop their goals and plans for getting from Here to There. It will be time well invested.

There's a difference between getting staff members the training they need to be compliant with regulations and getting them the training they need. Too often, caregivers show up for trainings with only one goal: to walk out of the room with a certificate that says they were present. I actually had a provider approach me once before a ninety-minute session on burnout and say, "I have to leave in fifteen minutes. Can I still get a sticker for my certificate to bring to my director?"

A better way is to work with your staff members to seek training they will find useful and interesting, that will inform them and help them do their jobs better. Sending staff members to training that they are not interested in, that they find meaningless, simply wastes time and resources. For budgetary reasons, directors too often seek out only those trainings that are nearby and inexpensive. They are more concerned about cost than quality. Find the right training, and staff members will walk away with more than a piece of paper to stuff in a file—they'll leave with new ideas and understanding, and they'll return to work energized, productive, and happy.

One of the major differences between a babysitter and an early care and education professional is training. When you force staff members to attend training that they find useless, unmotivating, and boring, you are doing nothing to build them up as professionals. In fact, you are hindering their professional growth. In too many programs, training and professional development is an afterthought. It falls far down the list of important concerns for too many directors. If you truly want to build an inspired and inspiring staff, you have to invest time and energy in meaningful training.

A Voice in Planning and Decisions

Offering staff members a voice in center operations is a great way to strengthen your team. It is not easy to do, but when staff members help to develop center policies and protocols, they are more apt to follow them. It would be very difficult to give your staff a voice in all decision making, and I suggest you start small. Next time you order books, equipment, or supplies, get the staff involved in selecting them. When you have a chance to renovate a classroom or the playground, form a committee of staff members to run the project. When they are ready for bigger challenges, assign them to revise your program fees or head lice policy. Giving staff members a real voice gives them power and ownership of the program. Environments where employees feel they have some control are less likely to cause burnout. Empowered employees with a sense of ownership are more productive and less likely to leave your program. Involving them in decision making takes some weight off your shoulders and encourages the leaders among them to emerge. It also provides you with an opportunity to break up your own routine.

Productive Meetings and Planning Time

If you are going to make room in the schedule and budget to pull your staff together for regular staff meetings—and I suggest that you do—make sure you are not wasting everyone's time. Make sure that the meetings are productive, succinct, and useful. People dislike feeling that their time is being squandered, and too many staff meetings leave them feeling that way.

Some tips for making meetings productive:

◄ Allow staff members to have input on the meeting's agenda.

◄ Make sure everyone gets a copy of the agenda at least forty-eight hours before the meeting.

◄ Be prepared. Have ready all the handouts and other supplies you will need.

◄ Start on time.

◄ Stay on task. Don't get sidetracked. If something unexpected comes up that needs to be discussed, table it until the next meeting.

◄ Finish on time.

Finding the time for planning is just as important as finding the time to hold regular meetings. If you want staff members to do their best possible work with the children, you have to give them time away from the kids to plan projects and activities. Staffers working with infants need this time as much as those working with preschoolers. Regular time each week is needed to prepare materials, build learning environments, gather supplies, think of activities, and develop goals. Like regular breaks, planning time is a challenge to budget and schedule for, but the payoff is higher quality care and a less stressed staff.

At least an hour of planning time a day would be great, but that is not always feasible. If you ask, I think you'll find that staff members without paid planning time would be ecstatic to get an hour a week.

Professional Relationships

It's hard to believe how many centers are infected with gossip, backstabbing, vindictiveness, deceit, and disingenuous behavior. Someone could write a soap opera: *As the Center Turns, Days of Our Day Care,* or *The Bold and the Bottle Fed.* I've heard stories about this stuff reaching the point where catfights break out *in the center.* Hair pulling, face scratching, down-to-the-floor brawls in front of children.

While fisticuffs are rare, the much more common two-faced behavior can get equally out of hand. Anything you can do to help build honest relationships with, and among, your staff helps diminish this playground behavior. Staff members do not have to be best friends or even like each other, but they do need to know how to work together in a professional manner. As a director, you can model this behavior; it's a way you can instill professional behavior in your staff.

Directors are often hurried, and this frequently means short, curt conversations with staff members, usually about problems or the trials and tribulations of the day. It is in your best interest to slow down and make time for pleasant conversation with your staff. Maybe you talk about the cute this-or-that that so-and-so did the other day, or compliment the way a staffer handled a particular situation, or just chat about the weather or an upcoming vacation—anything that helps to develop a personal bond. Making time for simple conversation strengthens your relationships, forces you to slow down, and makes you more approachable when a problem comes up. It will take practice, but it will be well worth your effort.

Competitive Benefits

Most providers who leave the child care profession say they do so because of poor benefits. One action you can take to cut down on burnout and turnover is to provide the best possible wages and benefits. I know from experience that the dollars to do this are somewhere between difficult and impossible to find, but the payoff is priceless. The quality of care goes up, turnover goes down, professionalism improves, and enrollment increases.

"What stresses you out about your job?" I asked a group of providers during a burnout training session. They called out some of the usual responses—for example, wages, parents, poor benefits, no breaks.

Then I noticed someone looking sheepishly from side to side, her neck craning to see if someone particular was in the room. When she realized it was safe to talk, she spoke, "I have this coworker who is driving everyone crazy. She . . ." What unfolded was an all-too-common story about a provider who managed to spread stress throughout an entire program; who raised blood pressures just by walking into the room; who prompted otherwise content people to dream of new jobs in happier work environments.

Sometimes such people are burned out and need to share

their troubles and frustrations with their coworkers. Other times, they simply have personalities that rub the majority of the staff the wrong way. Either way, one person can spread burnout through a center like head lice through a kindergarten class.

Anyone who has worked in a center-based program will probably recognize someone who has at least one of these traits:

- ◄ Incessantly complains about his work or home life

- ◄ Gossips and starts rumors

- ◄ Repeatedly misses work—usually on Mondays or Fridays (sometimes both in the same week)

- ◄ Has let his stress affect the quality of care he gives

- ◄ Is always late—for work, coming back from break, to staff meetings. The only time she is on time is to pick up her paycheck.

- ◄ Doesn't know he is burned out . . . but everyone who meets him does

- ◄ Knows she is burned out and feels that everyone she comes in contact with should share her pain

- ◄ Isn't qualified for the position he has or doesn't work well with children

- ◄ Knows everything about everything

Having one of these traits doesn't make a person a burnout version of Typhoid Mary; it simply makes him potentially annoying. However, two or more of these qualities means a good chance exists that a provider can spread burnout to everyone else she's exposed to. Such people whine, gossip, complain, irritate, bitch, and moan until coworkers want to string them up by their toes in retaliation. That might be a better response than what usually happens: in my experience, the response to these spreaders-of-burnout is that fellow staff members are usually polite to their faces and then complain about them behind their backs—either that, or they buy in to the complainer's feelings of discontent and become one of her followers.

I've seen these kind of people turn everyone in a center against them. Everyone on staff grows to despise such people and everything they say and do. Over time, the bad blood almost boils over. I've also observed them turn everyone against another person or policy when they start an uprising against a personal enemy or center policy they dislike. Others buy into the agitator's crusade, and all hell breaks loose. The power these people have has little to do with their personal shortcomings; it revolves around their ability to agitate and irritate. I don't have any idea of how to change these people—and that's not your responsibility. What you *can* do is keep your eyes open for the signs of infectious burnout from a problem employee. If you see it spreading, you can immunize yourself by not buying into the rabblerousing, then by opening honest lines of communications and continuing to seek opportunities to build a strong and honest relationship with this person. Part of what you need to communicate is that personal attacks are not among your center's values. You may want to provide training and opportunities for conflict resolution. In the end, if someone isn't willing to change, even after you've given her clear feedback on her behavior and the impact it's having on other staff members and provided her with opportunities to work things out, you may have to let her go.

Conclusion

You can use the steps outlined here to make center life better for caregivers. Implementing these steps will make your life as a director better too. You'll be happier at work, more productive, less stressed, and eager to take on new challenges when your coworkers are more in tune with their jobs.

JEFF A. JOHNSON, with his wife, Tasha, is the author of *Do-It-Yourself Early Learning: Easy and Fun Activities and Toys from Everyday Home Center Materials* (Redleaf Press, 2006). Jeff has sixteen years of experience as a community center and child care center director, and opened his own family child care program in 2003. He is a board member of the Iowa Association for the Education of Young Children and the National Association of Family Child Care and a frequent speaker on the topics of provider burnout and early learning at early childhood conferences around the country. His Web address is www.explorationsearlylearning.com.

Other Resources from Redleaf Press

DO-IT-YOURSELF EARLY LEARNING: EASY AND FUN ACTIVITIES AND TOYS FROM EVERYDAY HOME CENTER MATERIALS

Jeff A. Johnson & Tasha A. Johnson

 Written by two experienced child care providers, this book explains the construction and use of a variety of engaging, kid-tested play props, equipment, and activities that help children become more confident, stretch their intellect, and encourage play and exploration.

#107401-BR   **$19.95**

CELEBRATING YOUNG CHILDREN AND THEIR TEACHERS: THE MIMI BRODSKY CHENFELD READER

Mimi Brodsky Chenfeld

 Mimi Brodsky Chenfeld, a force of nature with fifty years of experience in the educational field, urges teachers to renew their spirits by reflecting on the magic of the classroom experience. Every page displays the warmth and wit that make Mimi beloved by early childhood professionals everywhere.

#537901-BR   **$14.95**

USE YOUR WORDS: HOW TEACHER TALK HELPS CHILDREN LEARN

Carol Garhart Mooney

 The connection between the ways we speak and the ways children behave and learn are examined in this humorous and thoughtful guide. Commonly missed opportunities to support cognitive development through meaningful conversation, develop receptive language and expressive language, and avoid and address behavioral issues in the classroom are reviewed.

#155401-BR   **$18.95**

FROM PARENTS TO PARTNERS: BUILDING A *FAMILY-CENTERED* EARLY CHILDHOOD PROGRAM

Janis Keyser

 From Parents to Partners explores how early childhood professionals can develop real partnerships with parents and other family members, as well as how to improve communication with them and give them a role to play in the organization—as members of curriculum committees, for example, or as teaching partners in the classroom.

#501401-BR   **$29.95**

Product availability and pricing are subject to change without notice.

800-423-8309 • www.redleafpress.org